Foreword

As the owner and founder of a number of medical spine pain clinics, I have treated and studied chronic spinal pain my entire professional career. Years ago there was very little clinical emphasis on the mind and body connection. Fortunately, that is changing. This book is based on good science, common sense and is a fascinating read.

Hypnosis can be a very helpful and effective option for patients who may not be responding to standard therapies. In fact, hypnosis can be used as an alternative to drug therapy to treat chronic pain. The type of hypnosis referenced in this book is safe, and comes without the negative side effects often seen with medication therapy, such as addiction. Ultimately, if patients can learn the techniques of self-hypnosis, they can reach the maximum benefit of mind and body balance.

Todd Ginkel, DC

Dedication

To all of my past clients, you have taught me valuable lessons in my life and career and I am in awe of the transformations you have made. I am honored to have been a part of your journey.

To all of my future clients, I look forward to assisting you in reaching your goals and I believe in your ability to realize the change you desire.

To all of you reading this book, I offer you confidence in your ability to break the bars of pain or whatever else might be standing in your way of the life you want. You have all you need to take back control.

Testimonials

"I had headaches every day for the past five years. Sometimes, they would get so bad I couldn't function for a few days. Practicing self-hypnosis has helped me manage my pain and stay calm and in control. I feel as though I have my life back again!" Katherine D., Chanhassen, MN

"I used hypnosis to prepare for a bi-lateral mastectomy. The surgery was a success and I used no pain meds as I felt only slight discomfort. A miracle? I don't think so. The positive thinking and intent prepared me and helped me through the process. I tell everyone I meet who is slated for surgery to try it." Victoria J., Tampa, FL

"I've had shoulder pain for years and take drugs to dull the constant pain. Hypnosis has helped me drastically reduce the number of meds I take, and I'm looking forward to eliminating them all together. It feels good to be taking control of my self again." Jack N., Burnsville, MN

"Fibromyalgia had greatly reduced the quality of my life. Now that I've learned techniques for managing my level of comfort, I'm sleeping at night and I feel calm and relaxed all over my body every day. A few short sessions and regular practice of self-hypnosis is all it takes!" Sherrill D., Eustis, FL

Table of Contents

Why You Should Read this Book   1
I Didn't Grow Up to Be a Hypnotist   3
Just the Facts   8
Pain and Painkillers   10
The Cost of Pain   14
Thinking Outside the Pill   16
Hypnosis – Not What You See in the Movies   21
Hypnosis is a Natural State of Mind   25
A Model of the Mind   30
The Four Laws of the Mind   33
Emotions and Pain   36
The Science Behind Hypnosis   43
The Pain is in Your Brain   46
Working with Clients   52
Your Autonomic Nervous System   55
It's All in Your Imagination   59
Just Breathe   61
Success Stories   64
Pain Studies on the Efficacy of Hypnosis   68
Choosing a Hypnotist   71
Parting Thoughts   74
About the Author   76
Citations   78
Gratitude   84

Why You Should Read this Book

This book is meant to educate you about the issues in our country related to pain and prescription pain medications like opioids. It is also meant to inform you of other alternatives to painkillers, in particular hypnosis, so you can make informed decisions about your healthcare. There are solutions for pain that don't have to be swallowed, inserted somehow into your body, or that don't have side effects. The "side effects" of painkillers can sometimes become worse than the original problem.

The information contained in this book comes from well-sourced, documented research and literature. It also comes from my own practical, real-life experience and the experiences of my clients.

Hypnosis is complementary to what you might already be doing to improve your physical, mental and emotional health. I work with doctors, psychologists and licensed therapists. The study of hypnosis is not included in their fields of study and so I find that the majority of them have little knowledge of how hypnosis works and the benefits their patients can receive. Perhaps this book will provide enough information to encourage healthcare providers to learn more about hypnosis, and to work in partnership with well-trained hypnosis professionals around the country.

What I have to say may never be popular. It may be written off and discarded by those who "know better." It's possible that my message will fall on the deaf ears of those who have too much to gain by maintaining the status quo.

In this world of twenty-four-hour news programs and the tremendous volume of "information" found online, it is sometimes hard to see the forest for the trees. And so, I write this book for two reasons:

> To let you know that you have more control over pain than you think you do.

> To educate you about hypnosis and its benefits in pain management.

I Didn't Grow Up to Be a Hypnotist

Hypnosis found me!

When I graduated high school in 1976, my teachers and guidance counselors advocated for a career in nuclear physics. Really! I still remember the drills where we would get under the desk and cover our heads. Even in fifth grade, I knew that was pretty dumb. For me, nuclear *anything* was never an option. I was awarded a full four-year scholarship to Northwestern to study English literature, and another to the University of Mexico to study Spanish (Knutson is my maiden name, by the way, so Spanish is not my native language). Bored with my private high school education, I said no to all of it.

I wanted to study something I knew nothing about, something that would excite me in a way high school never did. I landed at a local, now defunct college, studying fashion merchandising and business. Oh, boy. Fashion merchandising taught me to not care about what everyone else thought, and the business side really hooked me.

I've been a constant learner and entrepreneur my whole life. Give me something I don't know about and I'm all over it! I love the challenge of learning, building and succeeding.

My first "big girl" job in the late seventies was in sales and management in the male-dominated wine and liquor industry. I learned many life lessons. But with no future there, I started on my entrepreneurial track.

Thirty plus years later, I've run five successful business ventures as a: Certified Financial Planner, faux painting artist (while in the throes of early motherhood), founder and director of a Montessori school serving ages three to twelve, business consultant, and hypnotist. When I started these businesses, I knew absolutely nothing about any of them.

When I told people I was closing my sustainability consulting business to practice hypnosis, well, some thought I was crazy. But hypnosis is really not that different from the consulting I was providing at that time. I was teaching businesses about organizational change, systems thinking and how to sustain themselves for the long term. I now do this on an individual basis. I learned a long time ago that in order to make real change in an organization or in a community, you have to change the perspective of the individuals involved. It's what I've done in every one of my careers. I've just used different tools: money and planning, art and beauty, education and development, systems and planning, and now, with a tool that all of you have - the power of your very own subconscious mind!

In early 2013 I attended a retreat for personal growth and enjoyment. I was extremely impressed with the instructor and wanted to learn more from him. He taught only two classes a year, with limited students and a wait list a mile long. He used hypnosis, and so I thought that if I was to ever have a chance of getting into his class, I'd better learn how to "do" hypnosis. I found a hypnosis class and enrolled immediately - once again having no knowledge of what I was going to be studying. I was the only one in the class who had no intention of being a hypnotist.

At the same time I had been struggling for years with severe knee pain (due to cartilage loss) and was having difficulty with simple tasks, like walking around the grocery store. The pain had reduced my quality of life significantly and my only option seemed to be full knee replacements. After a couple of intriguing classes, the skeptic in me decided to put hypnosis to the test. I asked the instructor if hypnosis could get me out of pain. He said if I really wanted to get rid of the pain, anything was possible.

In just a few sessions I was pain free for the first time in years! The skeptical part of me was convinced. As I practiced the skills I was learning, I witnessed firsthand the benefits of hypnosis. I started working with people at home to refine my practical skills and to acquire more knowledge

The pills I didn't take!

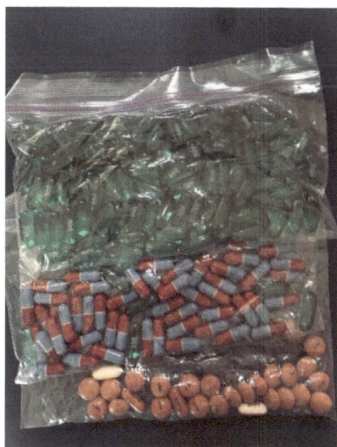

A year later, I decided to undergo a full bi-lateral knee replacement. Though I was no longer experiencing the pain I once had, my knees were structurally unsound (I kept falling down the stairs). I opted to have both knees replaced at the same time – one surgery, one general anesthesia, one rehab. After the surgery, I used self-hypnosis to control my pain instead of taking painkillers. While I was open to taking pain medications if necessary, I found that I didn't need them! During my six-week recovery, I estimate that I did without approximately 180 pills.

During my two-week stay at the rehabilitation center, I realized that hypnosis could be of value to all of the (mostly) older people who were there. Their issues - sleep, fear, confidence and pain - could all be improved using hypnosis. I felt compelled to provide the benefits of hypnosis to as many people as possible. I made the commitment then and there that I would sign a lease for office space the first day I could drive again.

I've never looked back. I started with a one-room office in a bank building. In October of 2015, I expanded to a 2,700 square foot facility, The FARE Hypnosis Center in Eden Prairie, Minnesota. The Center has offices for four hypnotists and a training center. I conduct classes and workshops open to the public, and train medical professionals and new hypnotists.

Now in my fourth year of practice, I am a Board Certified Hypnotist through the National Guild of Hypnotists (NGH) and a Certified Instructor. I am also a Certified Professional Hypnosis Instructor with the Banyan Hypnosis Center, the only other Guild certified program in the world. At this printing, I have more than 800 hours of training.

I didn't grow up to be a hypnotist - it found me, and it literally changed my life. I have seen transformational changes in clients on a wide variety of issues: sleep, fears, weight, smoking cessation, changing habits, building confidence. But some of the most satisfying clients I have worked with have been those dealing with pain.

Pain affects everything - mood, relationships, careers, family, finances, self-esteem and confidence - just to name a few. Pain creates stress, and stress creates more pain - a vicious cycle that *can* be broken or modified. As a systems thinker, I recognize the human mind and body as a system that can manifest many unexpected consequences when pain is present. When I can teach a client how to turn down the volume or eliminate pain, the consequences of that relief are far-reaching and extremely rewarding for both of us. I am in awe of what can transpire within my clients - what they are capable of accomplishing, ***simply with the skills and capacity they were given at birth.***

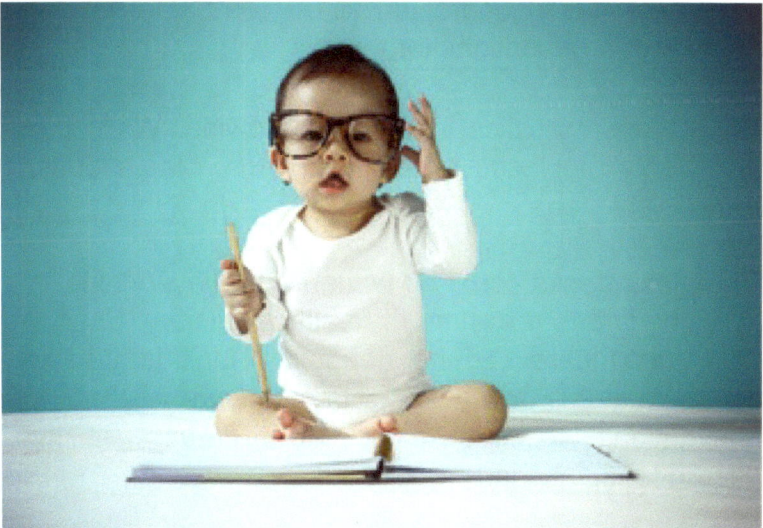

Before I address how hypnosis works, I want to be clear about why this issue of pain is so important.

Just the Facts

You can hardly pick up a periodical or go online these days without seeing something written about the enormous problems of prescription painkillers. As a hypnotist who understands the importance of words, I do not use the word "enormous" lightly. It only takes five short sentences to confirm why it is an appropriate word:

Chronic pain affects an estimated 100 million people - nearly *one - third* of our entire population. This is more than those affected by heart disease, diabetes and cancer combined.[1] Seventy-eight Americans die **every day** from an overdose of opioids. This includes heroin and prescription painkillers like oxycodone, hydro-codone and methadone. Deaths from prescription painkillers have quadrupled since 1999,[2] as have the number of prescriptions for them.[3]

I find these statistics to be mind blowing. While there are plenty of places to lay the blame, blame doesn't provide solutions.

Countless books could be written about everything that is wrong with our system of healthcare today. Even the word *healthcare* can be debated - isn't it "disease" care? I say this not to judge. I only desire to challenge conventional thinkers to be more creative in their search for solutions.

I am acutely aware of the complexity, challenges and unexpected consequences of changing our massive healthcare system. The relationship between hospitals,

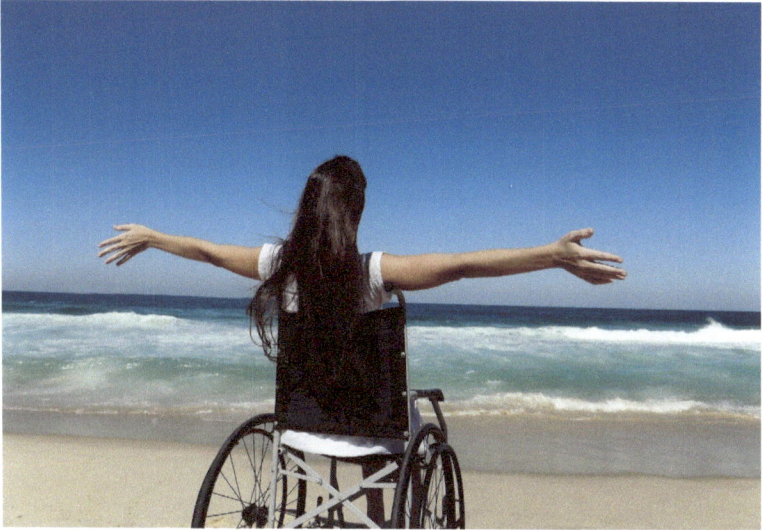

pharmaceutical companies, doctors, patients and insurers, and the scope of the issues involved with them are well beyond my pay grade. But that doesn't mean that any of us should hesitate to seek answers to the real problems we all face.

Pain and Painkillers

Americans are dealing with many types of acute and chronic pain. Acute pain can become chronic, and it's the chronic pain that often gets people hooked on drugs. The fact of the matter is that the body *heals* after injury or surgery. The time needed for the body to heal may vary, but the body *does* heal. Chronic pain is what exists after everything that can be done has been done. Pain does not always serve a purpose, as I will discuss shortly.

The four most common areas of chronic pain are:
- Low back pain (27%)
- Severe headache or migraine (15%)
- Neck pain (15%)
- Facial ache or pain (4%)

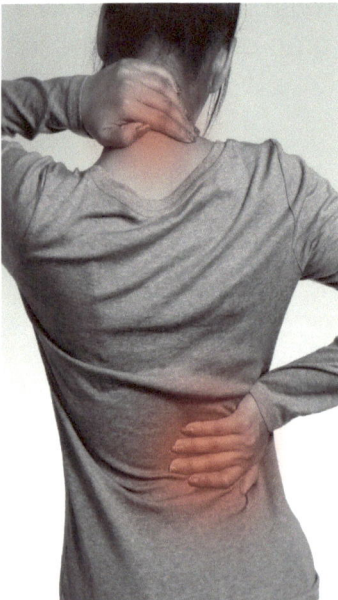

Back pain is the leading cause of disability in individuals under age forty-five. More than 26 million people between the ages of twenty and sixty-four have experienced frequent back pain. Low back pain greatly impacts the physical and mental health of those who suffer from it. 28% of adults with low back pain report limited activity due to a chronic condition, as compared to 10% of adults who do not have low back pain.

Also, adults reporting low back pain were three times as likely to be in fair or poor health, and more than four times as likely to experience serious psychological distress compared to those without low back pain.[4]

Usually the first line of treatment for low back pain, neck pain, and headaches is to prescribe some type of opioid. The opioid problem in the United States is serious. More people died from drug overdoses in 2014 than in any year on record and 60% of those deaths involved an opioid. Since 1999, the amount of prescription opioids sold in the United States nearly quadrupled; yet there has not been an overall change in the amount of pain that Americans report.[5-7]

If these statistics aren't enough to be concerned about, consider the following:

- Prescription drugs are the second-most abused category of drugs in the United States, following marijuana.[8]
- Among twelfth graders, pharmaceutical drugs used non-medically are six of the ten most-used substances. Nearly one-third (29%) of people age twelve or older who used illicit drugs for the first time in the past year began by using prescription drugs non-medically.[8,9]
- In 2009, the number of first-time, non-medical users of psychotherapeutics (prescription opioid pain relievers, tranquilizers, sedatives and stimulants) was about the same as the number of first-time marijuana users.[10]
- Of the 21.5 million Americans twelve or older that had a substance use disorder in 2014, 1.9

million involved prescription pain relievers and 586,000 involved heroin.[10]

- Four out of five new heroin users started out misusing prescription painkillers. As a consequence, the rate of heroin overdose deaths nearly quadrupled from 2000 to 2013. During this fourteen-year period, the rate of heroin overdose showed an average increase of 6% per year from 2000 to 2010, followed by a larger average increase of 37% per year from 2010 to 2013.[11]
- 94% of respondents in a 2014 survey of people in treatment for opioid addiction said they chose to use heroin because prescription opioids were "far more expensive and harder to obtain."[12]

There are many other statistics to add to this, but I think I've made my point.

Despite rising concerns about opioids, they are still the leading treatment for pain. In 2012, doctors in the United States wrote 259 million prescriptions, which is more than enough to give every American adult their own bottle of pills.[13]

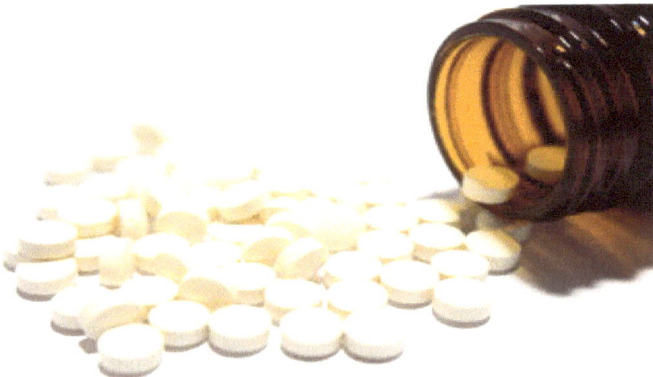

Though these drugs have been shown to be effective in treating pain, there has been little research on the long-term effects of continued use. A new study raises the concern that these drugs actually could *extend* chronic pain. The University of Colorado Boulder found evidence in rats that painkillers prolonged chronic pain by increasing the release of pain signals in the spinal cord.[14]

And yet, despite all of these concerns, answers to the issue of chronic pain and the opioid problem seem to focus only on the development of new kinds of drugs.

The Cost of Pain

In 2010, the annual cost of treating and managing pain in the United States was estimated to be between $560 billion and $635 billion. This includes the medical costs of care and the economic costs due to disability days, lost wages and productivity.[15]

In addition, it is estimated that the non-medical use of opioid pain relievers costs insurance companies up to $72.5 billion annually in healthcare costs.[16]

Back pain alone dramatically impacts productivity in the workplace. The Integrated Benefits Institute (IBI) is a leading workforce health and productivity research and measurement organization. According to their research, nearly one in four employees report experiencing low back pain. This costs employers $51,400 annually per 100 employees in medical treatments and lost productivity. Lost work time and underperformance at work (presenteeism) due to low back pain costs employers another $34,600 per 100 workers.[17]

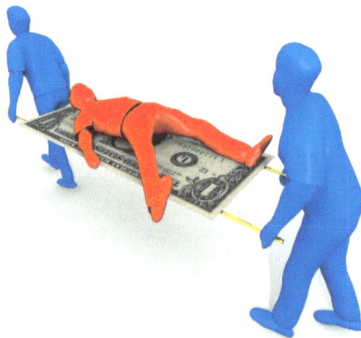

And of course, the unquantifiable but enormous cost of chronic pain and the opioid problem is the financial and emotional toll on relationships and families. It can affect the everyday lives of people in heart-wrenching ways.

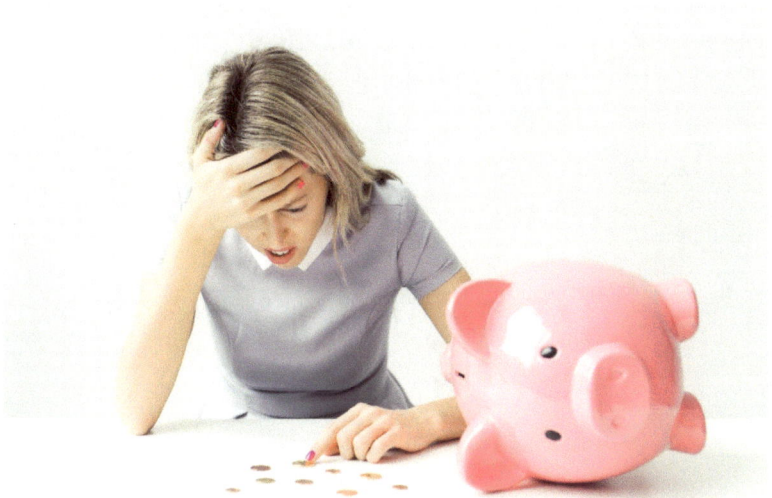

Thinking Outside the Pill

Prescription medications can play an important role in improving and maintaining your health, as can many procedures and practices in Western medicine. I believe there are other treatment options that can also be of value, even though they may or may not have scientifically proven research behind them.

Medical professionals are experts at what they do in their particular field, and are not necessarily aware or up-to-date about what other practitioners do in theirs. This can make it challenging for you to get information outside of what your current healthcare providers know. The Internet can prove helpful, overwhelming or

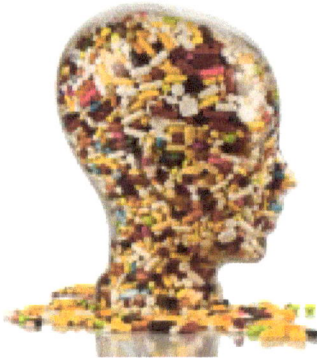

detrimental, due to the massive amounts of information it contains; and the difficulty in knowing what is truthful and accurate and what is not can be especially challenging. The numerous types of alternative options for relieving pain may also confuse you.

There are many researchers striving to understand our mind and bodies in greater detail in order to develop better approaches to healthcare. There are also alternative avenues to take when it comes to choosing your healthcare modalities. Some of these avenues don't require implanting or swallowing anything that might have adverse or negative consequences. Hypnosis is one of those options. But before I talk about hypnosis, I would like to mention other alternative modalities in general.

I am not an authority on these options, and so I cannot speak to any science or disclaimers associated with them, or their efficacy. However, some of these modalities have been around for a long time and are supported by anecdotal evidence:

Acupuncture has its roots in traditional Eastern Chinese medicine. The most common application for acupuncture is to reduce pain. Traditionally it is a technique to balance the flow of energy in the body, known as *qi* or *chi*. Practitioners of *Western* medicine believe acupuncture points are places that stimulate nerves, muscles and connective tissue, and can perhaps increase blood flow to stimulate the body's natural painkillers.

Chiropractic adjustment applies a controlled, sudden force to a spinal joint, called spinal manip- ulation. Its purpose is to correct structural alignment, reduce nerve irritation and improve bodily functions. It is commonly used to reduce back and neck pain and headaches.

Massage is a general term that has many different forms for pressing, rubbing and manipulating the skin, muscles, tendons and ligaments. Studies demonstrate that it is effective in reducing stress, pain and muscle tension.

Homeopathy is the treatment of disease by administering minute doses of natural substances that in a healthy person would produce symptoms of disease. Homeopathy is holistic because it treats the person as a whole. The homeopathic practitioner finds the homeopathic remedy that is most similar to that of the patient's physical, psychological and emotional characteristics and complaints. Then a homeopathic prescription is given to the patient to stimulate his/her own being, using an absolute minimal dosage.

Meditation is a word that has come to be used loosely in the modern world. There are many variations on how to practice it. Some people use the word to mean a time of contemplating or thinking; others use it to refer to daydreaming or fantasizing. In traditional meditation, the mind is clear and alert and inwardly focused, with the goal of silencing the mind. Some research points to the effectiveness of meditation for stress and an improvement of overall health. While hypnosis and meditation may appear to be similar, there are some distinct differences, especially in the area of intention.

It's important to talk with your doctor about alternative modalities you may wish to try. Their knowledge and advice is an important piece of the larger puzzle that you can use to become an informed consumer and to make the best decisions for yourself. Your goal should be to determine what seems reasonable and logical to you, and to test and evaluate what feels right and produces the best results.

Federal and state governments are starting to address the opioid issue. The Centers for Disease Control and Prevention (CDC) has guidelines for doctors for prescribing painkillers and there are a few states that have done the same. The state of Ohio's Opiate Action Team suggests hypnosis as a non-pharmacologic treatment. Hopefully, other states will follow suit.

Ohio's Guidelines for the Management of Acute Pain Outside of Emergency Departments

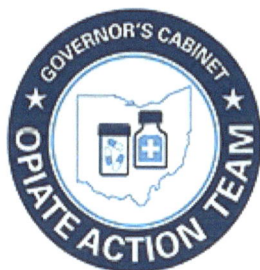

Non-Pharmacologic therapies should be considered as first-line therapy for acute pain unless the natural history of the cause of the pain or clinical judgment warrants a different approach. These therapies often reduce pain with fewer side effects and can be used in combination with non-opioid medications to increase likelihood of success. Examples may include, but are not limited to:
- Ice, heat, positioning, bracing, wrapping, splints, stretching and directed exercise available through

physical therapy
- Massage therapy, tactile stimulation, acupuncture/acupressure, chiropractic adjustment, manipulation and osteopathic neuromuscular care
-Biofeedback and **hypnotherapy**

Albert Einstein said, "We cannot solve our problems with the same thinking that we used when we created them." Perhaps this is true with the way we look at pain and the opioid problem. Replacing drugs with other kinds of drugs may or may not be the solution. We spend well over $1 trillion every year in the healthcare Industry. It is a complex system that cannot change on a dime. However, Einstein defined insanity as doing the same thing over and over again and expecting different results. Is it time to think and do things differently?

And this brings us to the topic of *hypnosis*, which is a subject that I am qualified to speak to you about in depth. Here is what hypnosis can do for you:

**You can manage your own pain
independent of anyone else,
with no ongoing costs
and with no negative side effects,
once you've
learned self-hypnosis.**

Hypnosis - Not What You See in the Movies

You follow the swinging watch and the next thing you know you are robbing a bank. You look into his eyes and divulge all of your secrets. A stranger whispers in your ear "Sleep!" and you fall under her spell. You read a book and are programmed to buy another copy of *Catcher in the Rye*.

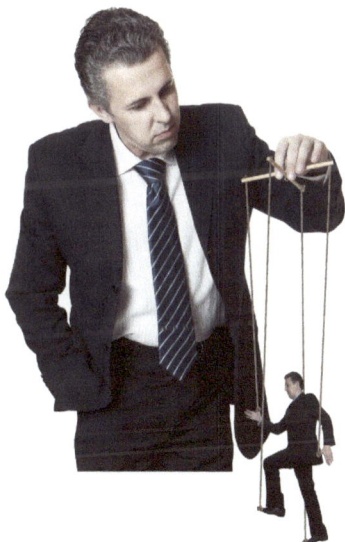

Like the soon-to-be-victim who doesn't turn on the lights or run out of the house when she thinks something is wrong, these scenarios make for good movies or television shows. But in reality, if I had that kind of power as a hypnotist, I wouldn't have to be writing this book, and we most certainly would not have a problem with opioids!

Here are the facts: hypnosis is a 100% consent state - I cannot hypnotize you if you don't want to be hypnotized. You won't do something that is against your will or morals. You can emerge from hypnosis whenever you want. I don't have any special powers.

I'm not psychic. I cannot guarantee anything. I can't *make* you go into a trance, but you *can* be hypnotized. There is only a small percentage of the population that can't be hypnotized. The main reason someone can't be hypnotized is because he or she doesn't want to be. I remind those clients who say that they can't give up control that they are actually more in control while in trance than in their normal conscious state, because in trance they are using the most powerful part of their mind.

The most frequent question I am asked is "How many sessions will it take for me to achieve my goal?" Although I can give you guidelines, I really don't know until we start working together. On average, clients usually fall into one of two categories: four one-hour visits or six two-hour visits. Some clients need less time, some need more. I teach every client self-hypnosis so he or she can be empowered to keep control of his or her own life. Once we are done working together, people rarely need to come back if they continue to practice the techniques they learned. Keep in mind that other hypnotists may employ other techniques, so their processes may vary from mine.

What determines if hypnosis works for you? You don't have to believe that hypnosis will work, but you DO have to *want* the change you seek. I tell clients that I am like a bicycle - I can transport you in the direction of your goals, but *you* have to peddle and *you* have to steer. I have no magic wand, no silver bullet.

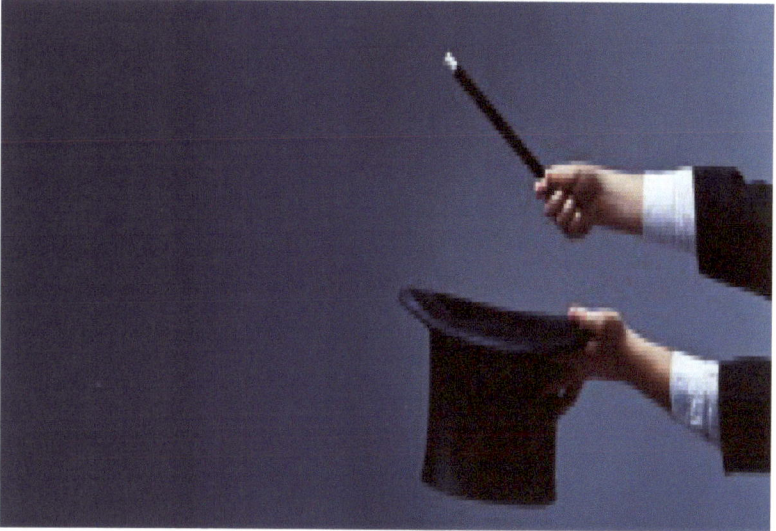

Like most things in life, you will get out of this process what you put into it. Most of the tools you have used to try to solve your problems have been done with the conscious mind. The thing that makes hypnosis different is that it works with your *subconscious* - the most powerful part of your mind. Hypnosis helps you use the power of your mind to reach your goals in the way that is best for you.

I don't have any of your answers. *You* do. **You came into this life with everything you need to do exactly what you were meant to do.** The one thing that I am absolutely certain of is that your subconscious mind knows exactly what your problems are, and it knows how to solve them. I simply facilitate your discovery of those things.

Drugs don't heal you. Doctors don't heal you. I don't heal you. Your body, and if you so believe, your Higher Power, heals you. Drugs, doctors, hypnosis and other alternatives simply help improve the environment for your body to do the work it is designed to do.

If you want it.

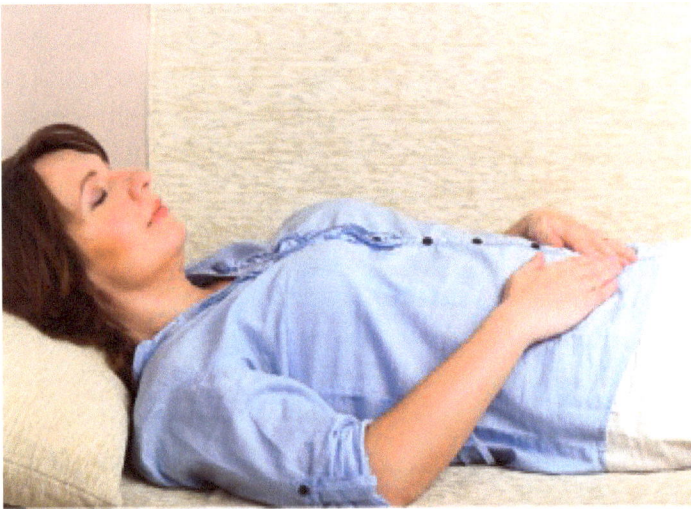

Hypnosis is a Natural State of Mind

There are several definitions of hypnosis. The official government definition is "the bypass of the critical factor of the conscious mind (that judgment part of ourselves), and the establishment of acceptable selective thinking."[18] The definition I prefer is "a state of heightened awareness and focused attention, where the individual is open to new thoughts and ideas." I cannot "put" you into the trance state. I simply serve as a guide and facilitator.

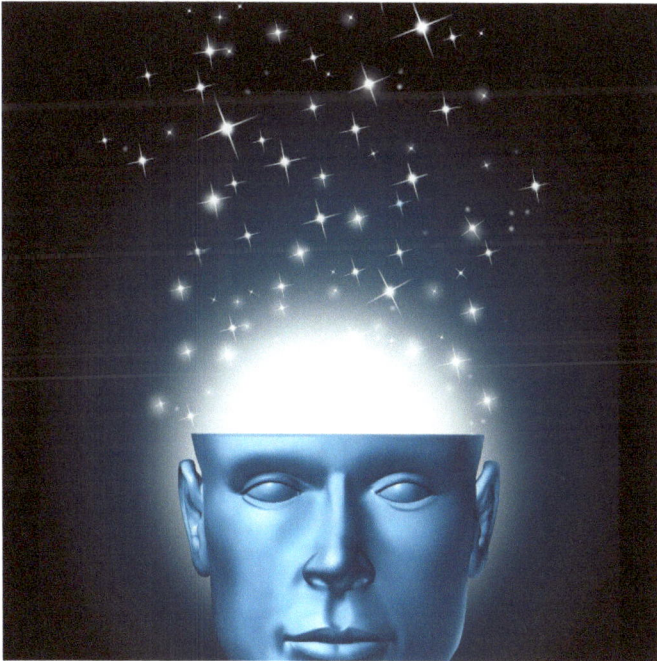

Hypnosis is a natural state of mind. You go in and out of hypnosis at least twice every day - when you pass through the alpha and theta trance states as you wake in the morning, and as you fall asleep at night. In hypnosis, the electrical activity patterns in your brain change, and they are measured in hertz (abbreviated Hz). Trance is a chemical reaction that happens in your brain. As such, sometimes there is a formal induction, as when working with a hypnotist, and at other times it is self-induced, intentionally or not.

States of Consciousness

Beta – The conscious mind is functioning; 13 to 30 Hz

Alpha – The day dreaming state; 8 to13 Hz

Theta/Trance – This is where you can change the conversation in your mind because you have full access to your imagination; 4 to 8 Hz

Delta – You are sleeping; 0 to 4 Hz

Trance that occurs during the daytime is typically a light, alpha trance state. The phenomena of driving from one place to another and not remembering how you got there is called Highway Hypnosis. To some degree your conscious mind checks out and the subconscious mind takes over, getting you there safely.

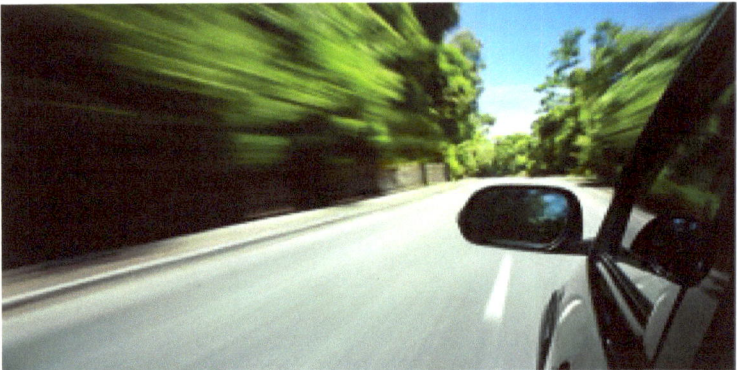

Trance can happen while reading a book, watching television or a movie, working, gardening, cooking, or any other activity in which you engage your concentration to the exclusion of everything else. If your attention is needed elsewhere, your subconscious mind directs you to that place. When you emerge from trance, you are often surprised to see how much time has passed without an awareness of that time passing.

Many aspects of the hypnotic state have been studied to answer questions such as:
- Is it sleep?
- Is the person just following instructions or otherwise making things up?
- Is it a placebo?

Here are some results from studies that have been conducted to address these questions:

The word *hypnosis* is of Greek origin and means "sleep." For a long time it was thought that hypnosis was a sleep state. Various studies have been conducted to determine whether hypnosis is a separate state distinct from sleep, an altered state, or if the person is simply complying with the hypnotist's instructions.[19] In a study published in *The American Journal of Psychiatry*, hypnosis was induced in participants who were then scanned with positron emission tomography (PET). The color perception areas of their cerebral hemispheres were activated when they were given the suggestion to see color, whether they were looking at color or black-and-white patterns. When they were given the suggestion to see black and white, the color perception areas of the brain showed decreased activity regardless of what the subjects were viewing. This implies that hypnosis is not a process of simply following instructions, but actually involves a change in the brain's perception.[20, 21] This is an important point to remember when I talk later about how clients can change their perception of pain while in hypnosis.

Hypnosis is not a state of sleep or relaxation. I use relaxation in hypnosis because it feels good for the client, and it is especially helpful in allowing a client with pain to escape from uncomfortable feelings. But hypnosis doesn't have to involve relaxation. Watch a hypnosis stage show and you'll see participants in everything but a relaxed state! In another study, volunteers underwent hypnotic induction with use of either the traditional method involving progressive relaxation or other classical techniques. In other volunteers hypnosis was induced by an active, alert method involving riding a stationary bicycle while receiving suggestions for alertness and activity. Equally receptive trance states were achieved by the relaxation and the alert methods.[22,23] There have been times when I have been talking with a client at my desk and the client became emotional I can induct her simply by asking her to close her eyes because emotion can induce trance. If I have given my client a post-hypnotic suggestion for induction in a previous session, trance can be instantaneous without relaxation of any kind.

A Canadian study with hypnotized persons showed the activation of a region in the right anterior cingulate cortex, an area that becomes activated when sound is heard or when sound is suggested (or hallucinated) in hypnosis, but not when sound is simply imagined. This implies that the mind registered the hypnotic hallucination as if it were real.[24] This illustrates an important distinction in the effectiveness of suggestions given in hypnosis, where the subconscious mind is actively engaged in hallucinating, instead of simply repeating affirmations using the conscious mind.

Like this Canadian study, there have been numerous neuroscience experiments that have shown that the brain cannot tell the difference between what is real, and what is vividly imagined or emotionally felt. Imaging techniques, like fMRI (functional magnetic resonance imaging), show that some of the same areas of your brain that process thoughts (for example, when I think about moving my finger), also process the actual behavior (for example, when I actually move my finger).

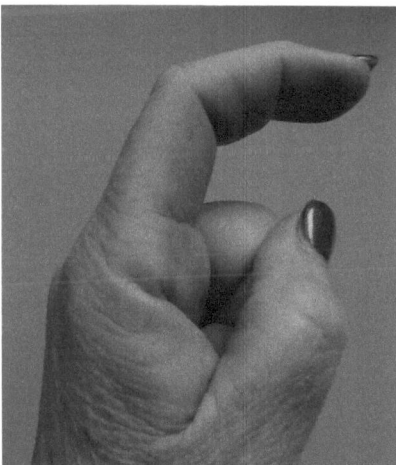

Neuroscientists Guang Yue and Kelly Cole conducted a study that looked at two groups over four weeks; group one exercised a finger, and group two *imagined* exercising the finger. In the end, the group that had actually performed the finger exercise, had increased strength of 30 Group two, that had only *imagined* exercising the finger, had increased strength of 22%[25]

A Model of the Mind

To understand hypnosis, let me give you a greatly simplified look at how your mind works by introducing four concepts: the conscious mind, the unconscious mind, the subconscious mind, and the critical factor.

The conscious mind is home to logic, ideas, willpower, affirmations, short-term memory and all of your "shoulds." Approximately 5% of your processing ability occurs in the conscious mind. On your best day you can work with only about seven to nine things at a time before you start to get overwhelmed, or things start falling through the cracks.

The unconscious mind is home to the regulation of your bodily processes, such as regulating your heartbeat and your breathing. The subconscious mind houses your imagination, rules, emotions, beliefs, values, filters, long-term memory, life stories, intuition and your "wants." Approximately 95% of your processing power occurs in these two parts of your mind. The subconscious mind shapes 95% or more of your life experiences.[3]

Then there is your brain's protective mechanism, the critical factor. The critical factor begins to form around the age of seven or eight, during the time when the logical part of your mind is forming. It continues forming into your teen years. The critical factor blocks instant communication from the subconscious to the conscious mind to protect you from overload. It can censor or judge ideas and thoughts that may be contrary to beliefs, rules or emotions that are held in your subconscious mind.

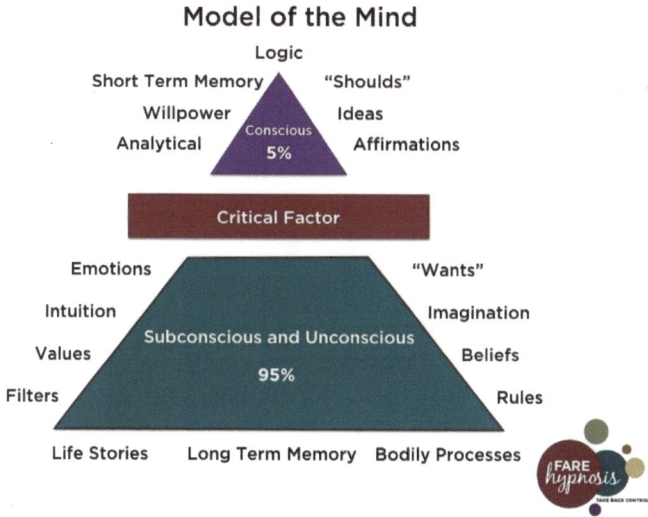

Model of the Mind

Logic

Short Term Memory   "Shoulds"

Willpower   Ideas

Analytical   **Conscious 5%**   Affirmations

Critical Factor

Emotions   "Wants"

Intuition   Imagination

Values   **Subconscious and Unconscious 95%**   Beliefs

Filters   Rules

Life Stories   Long Term Memory   Bodily Processes

FARE *hypnosis*
FARE BACK CONTROL

It is important to remember that:

- Most of your life stories and beliefs are given to you before the critical factor is formed - when you believed in Santa Claus and had no life experience or logic of your own.
- The critical factor opens to some degree when you are in the theta state so that the information stored there can be accessed.
- The alpha trance state is your mental escape or recharge that gives your conscious mind a rest when it is feeling over-loaded or over-processed.
- In trance, you are more in control because you are using the most powerful part of your mind, the subconscious.

Your subconscious mind retains memories and emotions throughout your life. Most likely you don't have many memories before the age of five. This is because the critical factor is protective and helps maintain order of those experiences. Imagine taking that pyramid of the model of the mind, and turning it upside down, like a funnel. If your protective mechanism, the critical factor wasn't in place, your "library" of information, emotions, experiences and memories that is stored in your subconscious mind would overwhelm your weaker conscious mind.

The downside to the critical factor is that memories, emotions, and beliefs that are stored in the subconscious mind cannot be easily accessed using the conscious mind. It is in the trance state that the subconscious mind can be accessed, and beliefs and rules that no longer serve you can be changed.

The Four Laws of the Mind

The first thing I learned in class about hypnosis was the Four Laws of the Mind. They so easily sum up the concepts, process and effects of hypnosis, that I named my business after their acronym - FARE.

Focus

Whatever you focus on will expand in your life. When the same behaviors keep producing the same results that you don't want, it's time to look at what your mind is focusing on. We focus on solutions.

Associate

When your thoughts and images are similar in nature to your focus, your mind begins to connect everything to that focus. We help eliminate triggers that reinforce unwanted behaviors.

Repeat

Whatever you repeat often enough, and believe passionately enough, will become the truth in your mind. We make sure your beliefs are aligned with your goals.

Expect

You get exactly what you expect you will, and your subconscious mind will filter out anything to the contrary. We align your expectations with your goals.

These laws of the mind, along with what is known about the model of the mind, make hypnosis a very powerful tool in affecting change.

As a hypnotist,

I focus on solutions. What you think about expands and manifests. If you are focusing on negative things - and most people do exactly that - I help you reframe the negatives in a positive way. The positive is what you actually want, not what you don't want. The subconscious mind doesn't understand sarcasm or negatives, and it is very literal. So if you are thinking, "I never think about my pain," it will hear "I think about my pain."

I help you eliminate triggers. I address habits of thoughts and behaviors and what triggers them in order to find the best avenues for change. For example, a golfer who gets out his water ball when he approaches the lake is giving himself the powerful suggestion that he will hit the ball into the water. In the same way, you make similar suggestions about how you will feel pain. You may have had to park far away from the door of the grocery store and your back felt pain by the time you got inside. So now you circle the parking lot again and again until you find a "close enough" spot. Or perhaps you carry your handicap tag with you when you ride in someone else's car "just in case" you can't find a close enough spot. The handicap tag becomes your water ball and is now associated with your pain. It has become a trigger for that thought or behavior.

I make sure your beliefs are aligned with your goals. When there is an emotional or physical trauma, it is easy to form powerful beliefs around it. Initially these beliefs may have served you well, but as your body heals, they may no longer be necessary. Because your mind always has the goal of keeping you safe it hangs on to those old habits and thoughts, impeding your healing.

I make sure your expectations are aligned with your goals. Your critical factor, the protective part of your mind, keeps out anything contrary to your expectations, even if they are outdated or misinformed. You will get exactly what you expect you will get.

Addressing any of these four laws can initiate life-altering changes.

Emotions and Pain

A computer is a good metaphor for how the Four Laws and the model of your mind interact. Your subconscious mind is like a hard drive with endless storage capacity. It's the storage place for your memories of experiences, emotions and beliefs. You don't even know most of what is there because it stays quiet, behind the scenes - like cookies left from websites you visit, or software that you installed years ago but no longer use. None of these things cause problems until one day, you install some new software, or you get a virus from something you downloaded. Things start to go haywire - maybe slowly at first, maybe instantly.

You enlist that awesome, logical and analytical conscious mind to solve the problem. But your conscious mind can't figure it out, because it doesn't understand the problem or it isn't experienced with solving the problem. But your mind discovers a work-around. It creates distractions such as cleaning your keyboard or rebooting frequently. And the distractions actually work...for a while.

Unfortunately, the real problem has never been solved. That virus, or those software conflicts keep growing, and before long they freeze your computer. Now you've got to take it to a computer specialist and that is going to cost you! The cost is not just monetary; you've also lost time and productivity. And if it's really bad, you've lost data.

You beat yourself up because you *know* that you shouldn't have ignored the problem, and now you are very frustrated with your computer. Maybe you just give up, or find more powerful distractors like using your tablet or phone, and you ignore the problem even longer. Perhaps the specialist finally suggests that it's time to get a new computer.

This is where the metaphor has to end. We only have one body and one mind, and they have to serve us for the rest of our lives.

There is a powerful mind-body connection. You know your thoughts become things. Your thoughts create real emotions, feelings and behaviors. It's time to dive a little deeper and look at emotions, because they play a role in your experience of pain, and your health in general.

The Secret Language of Feelings, by Calvin Banyan, MA, BCH, explains how emotions and feelings manifest in your body. First there is perception - what is detected through the senses. What you perceive interacts in the

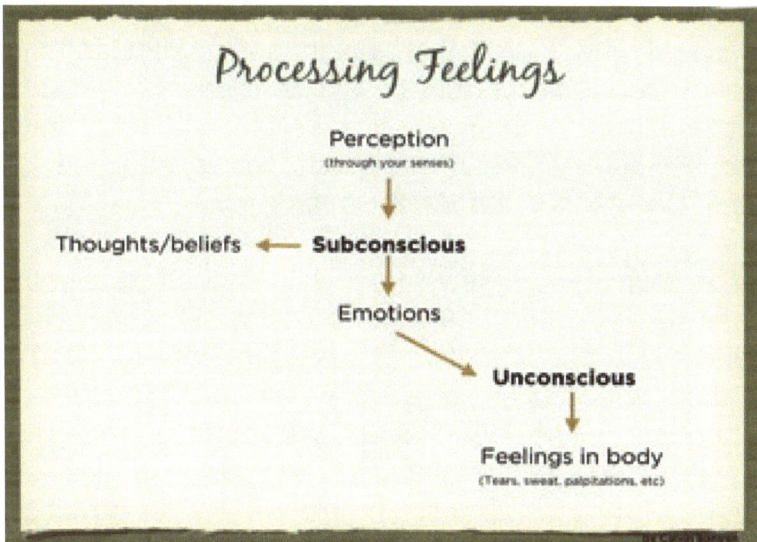

Processing Feelings

Perception
(through your senses)

↓

Thoughts/beliefs ←— **Subconscious**

↓

Emotions

↘

Unconscious

↓

Feelings in body
(Tears, sweat, palpitations, etc)

subconscious mind with your beliefs, creating an emotion. This emotion is not recognized in the conscious mind until the unconscious mind generates a feeling in your body. For example, fear might produce sweat; sadness might generate tears; worry might make your heart beat faster. Negative emotions are a warning sign that there is a need, want or desire that is not being met. All emotions are good. They tell you to pay attention so you can provide a satisfying response.[33]

Banyan compares emotions to an illuminated oil light on the dashboard of your car. Something needs attention. And it's always better to pay for a quart of oil now than ignore it until it has affected many parts of your car's engine, resulting in a more expensive repair bill.

It is then, after the emotion is felt in the body as a physical feeling, that the conscious mind can connect to what is happening, and the conscious mind goes into *its* job of analyzing and trying to figure it out. But here's the problem: the job of the conscious mind is to be analytical and logical, to reason and understand. It cannot perform the job of the subconscious mind, whose job is to deal with the beliefs and rules that you've created, and the emotions you've attached to them. One cannot perform the other's job.

All of your life you have been told how to deal with those pesky, rotten emotions: "Keep a stiff upper lip." "It's not nice to get angry." "Crying is for babies." "Don't let them see you are afraid." "Be strong." "You're the man of the house." "Suck it up!" As you hear the voice of your parents and grandparents in your head, this list can go on and on. Emotional pain, as well as physical pain, can become a false badge of courage or strength.

You may not have been taught that all emotions are good, that they are simply a signal that something needs attention. Emotions may even make you feel uncomfortable. Instead of finding a satisfying response that is appropriate for the emotion, you may choose to use distractors to avoid them completely. You may use food, tobacco, over-working, alcohol, shopping, gambling or some other excessive behavior to help you avoid uncomfortable feelings and temporarily make you feel better.

It takes tremendous energy to suppress your emotions. Emotions are meant to be expressed, not kept inside of you. Sooner or later, they WILL manifest - emotionally or physically. As Henry Maudsley said, "Sorrow not vented in tears, can make your organs weep."

Medical professionals can attest to the number of times a patient will exhibit real, physical symptoms, but they cannot find a physiological cause for them. You may have been told that your pain or illness is all in your head, when in fact it may be all in the subconscious part of your mind that hasn't been allowed to properly understand or express the emotions you've been working so hard to ignore.

I see many clients who come in for one reason (for example, to quit smoking or lose weight) and while in hypnosis, find themselves identifying emotions they didn't know existed, with causes they were never even aware of. This happens frequently with chronic pain. *Emotions* **allow the** *feelings* **to continually manifest**

in the body as pain, when in fact the body has already been healed. Like emotions, pain is also a warning sign - that something is wrong and needs attention. But over time the body heals and in most cases, the pain *should* go away.

Though it didn't manifest in physical pain, I'll use myself as an example of how suppressed emotions can affect the body. About fifteen years ago, I became very ill with Graves' disease, an autoimmune thyroid disease (where the body attacks itself). With a resting heart rate of 142, I gained seventy pounds in five months and had symptoms in nearly every part of my body. I was experiencing something called "thyroid storm." My thyroid stimulating hormone (TSH) levels were 48 - the normal range is between 0.5 and 5. It took three months on medication to lower my marathon beating heart to 100, before they could safely irradiate my thyroid. It was another two years before I was stable on synthetic hormone medication. During that time, I continued to gain even more weight. Years later, though I had lost and regained some of the weight on several occasions, it just kept finding it's way back to me again.

The endocrinologist explained that Graves' disease is typically brought on by physical or emotional trauma. At the time, my conscious mind could not come up with a reason for why this could be happening. I felt that my body had betrayed me. It was much later, when I became a hypnotist, that I would understand that I had buried some intense emotional trauma that had occurred a few years prior to my illness. After using hypnosis to help me uncover the hurt and anger I still held inside, I came to realize the reasons I had been unable to get rid of the weight.

I'm now thirty pounds lighter, and I'm confident that these pounds shall not return. I am still on the journey with quite a few pounds left to shed. It's like peeling back the layers of an onion, complete with crying at times, but this time losing the weight has been easier. I have a different relationship with food and with my body, now that I understand my emotions. This time I know that the *real* work is being done. The weight and eating were simply distractors for the emotions I had kept hidden. In letting go of the beliefs and thoughts that no longer serve me, I am paving the way on my road to health.

While this part of my story did not manifest in physical "pain", the scenario is relevant to the topic of this book. The roots of my story are the same as those with the end result of chronic pain: emotions held in or stifled can manifest in all kinds of stress and physical problems.

And so, it is possible to perceive pain as a better option to an emotion you may not want to face or no longer understand or recognize. For example, a person whose injury leaves him unable to perform the job he loved and identified with may feel:
- Inadequate - There's nothing else I'm qualified to do.
- Sad - I've lost the ability to do what I value the most.
- Angry - It's not fair!
- Guilty - I can't support my family.

Perhaps he feels all of these emotions, and in addition, loneliness and boredom. Pain becomes *who he is.* It becomes his expectation.

A healthcare professional may have told you, "There is nothing else we can do for you. You'll just have to live with the pain." Your literal subconscious mind interprets that as "live with the pain or die." Though neither of those options is appealing, opting for the pain seems the lesser of two evils.

Let me end this chapter with another metaphor. When dealing with beliefs and emotions, hypnosis can be like cleaning your garage. You've packed a lot of stuff in there over the years, and now it's so full you can't drive the car in. You know where most of the important stuff is, but it's getting harder to get to it and you find yourself tripping over lots of stuff in the process. You decide it's time to clean out that garage before it's completely out of control. You take everything out into the driveway - sorting what goes to charity, what needs to be thrown out, what you are going to keep, and how it should be organized as it comes back into the garage. It's a lot of work, but it gives you a great feeling of accomplishment and satisfaction. Getting rid of that old, outdated and useless stuff has been worth the hard work. And you can even park the car inside again!

The Science Behind Hypnosis

We have known for a long time that hypnosis works. We have not always understood why or how. Today, with the advent of imaging techniques like fMRI and PET, the field of neuroscience allows us to observe and study what happens in the brain during the trance state. While there is still much we don't know, what we do know about what happens in the brain makes it possible for us to further improve and refine our hypnotic techniques. We also have learned that the brain is "plastic", meaning that it has the ability to change and reconfigure itself. This is very good news for those of us who want to think differently, change habits, feel better and change our perceptions about pain. You *can* teach an old dog new tricks!

There have been many clinical studies on hypnosis, especially regarding the impact of hypnosis in dealing with pain. In this book, I present some of the findings that are relevant to you as a consumer of healthcare. This will enable you to make more informed decisions and take responsibility for the management of your pain and overall health.

As a hypnosis practitioner, I want to offer a salient observation about the clinical trials and research on hypnosis. The gold standard of a randomized, double-blind, controlled trial is virtually impossible when studying the effects of hypnosis. Even the best studies may fail to assess the tangible impacts of hypnosis because of all the variables involved. Hypnosis is by no means a one-size-fits-all process. Factors that must be taken into consideration for hypnosis to be effective include:

- The participant's personality and characteristics
  - Are they analytical or imaginative?
  - How hypnotizable are they?
  - Are they comfortable with and do they understand the process and the suggestions?
  - How important are the benefits and outcomes of the hypnosis to them?
  - What is their level of skepticism in belief and willingness for the desired change?
- The rapport or lack of with the hypnotist
- The setting and stress level of the participant
- The techniques used and the delivery of the suggestions
- Depth of the trance state
- The length and number of sessions
- Follow-up and continuing practice of self-hypnosis

Because of all these variables, it is difficult to look at one individual study that pertains to a specific result in using hypnosis to address a particular issue. A better way, though still imperfect, is to measure overall results using meta-analysis, or averaging the results of many related studies that use similar techniques. More research is needed to help fortify the thousands of anecdotal cases involving hypnosis and medical and psychological issues.

Results from clinical trials may not accurately estimate the effectiveness achievable in an office setting with willing, expectant patients. In clinical trials, many patients are likely to be unwilling, unmotivated or skeptical about hypnosis. Hypnosis appears to be "particularly useful and yields better results when it is specifically requested by the patient. Consequently, clinical trials may underestimate the benefits of hypnosis compared with those obtainable by a proficient, experienced hypnotist."[22]

My experience indicates that the most successful clients are the ones with the greatest desire for change. I doubt that this fact is present in clinical trials and research. However, with all of this being said, it *is* important to evaluate results to the best of our ability, as it has been for me to satisfy my own particular need for documented "proof." (As if my own experience hasn't been enough!) After I have explained how pain is processed in the body, I'll provide information on some pain studies to help you become an even more informed consumer.

The Pain is in Your Brain

There are many misperceptions about the concept of pain. If you take nothing else away from this book, I hope it is this:

Pain is experienced based on your environment, emotions, previous experiences and perceptions, and your brain decides to what extent and how you feel it!

In this chapter, physical therapist and clinical neuroscience researcher Adriaan Louw, PhD provides a simplified explanation of how the pain process works in your body.[34]

Let's say you were crossing the street and you fell and badly sprained your ankle. You look up and see a bus coming and it can't stop before it runs over you. Your brain might perceive the bus as a bigger threat, so you would get up and run out of the way, feeling nothing of your badly sprained ankle. After you got to safety, the brain may then perceive the danger in your ankle and it would start to hurt.

There is no processing center in your brain for pain like there is for sight and hearing and language. Signals are sent from the injured area, letting the brain know that something is wrong. The brain then decides if there is a real danger, and what to do about it.

Have you ever woken up and found a big bruise on your body? You wonder how this could have happened without your knowledge. Your brain decided that what had happened wasn't a danger and didn't feel the need to let you become aware of it. It is also possible that you were in a trance state, so involved with what you were focused on at that moment that you tuned everything else out and simply didn't notice.

Pain can occur with or without injury or surgery. In fact, about 25% of people with pain have neither had injury or surgery. As we have already discussed, pain can stem from your emotions. The pain from the loss of a loved one or from cutting off your arm is processed the same way in your brain. It cannot differentiate between emotional or physical pain.

Your nerves have constant electrical currents running through them. The currents change with stress, movement, temperature, blood flow and many other factors. Your nerves have receptors and sensors in all of your tissues for many types of conditions, and they change depending on what is needed at the time. For example, when they feel cold air they make you more sensitive, reminding you to put on a sweater.

When the nerves in your tissues continually send danger messages (called nociception) to the spinal cord, a door opens to relay information to the brain. Over long periods, the system just leaves the door open wide so more information can be sent to the brain. You become so ultra sensitive that even a light touch may be sent on

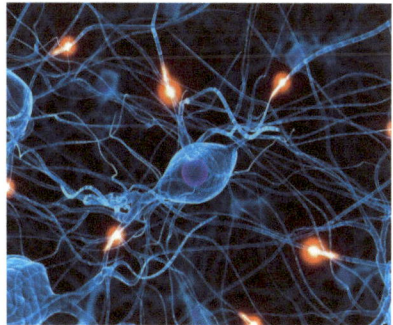

to the brain for interpretation. This is what happens when you have chronic pain. The pain you feel doesn't mean the tissue hasn't healed or that there is anything wrong, your nerves have just become more sensitive.

Your brain produces chemicals that are fifty times more powerful than any drugs you could take. When there is an injury, it produces chemicals, such as endorphins, that ease the incoming danger messages and "water down" the pain. Let's say you get up to go to the bathroom in the middle of the night and stub your toe. It really hurts. Your brain produces these calming chemicals, and when it determines that the injury doesn't require more serious attention, the pain begins to ease. By the time you get back to bed you hardly notice your toe.

With chronic pain, your brain takes away this natural medicine to protect you. It may seem counterintuitive, but it does this to make you *more* sensitive so you'll do something about it. This causes stress, and you feel even more pain when you are stressed. Your nerves go into an ultra sensitive feedback loop. This feedback loop can become a habit, and hypnosis can be very helpful in changing that habit.

You are constantly bombarded with ideas about how and what you should feel. Healthcare providers, television commercials, family and friends all provide input, and most of it is negative. It is very hard to have your *own* opinions with so much external input. You form beliefs based on other people's experiences and what you are told might happen, and this can create an expectation of what pain should feel like for you.

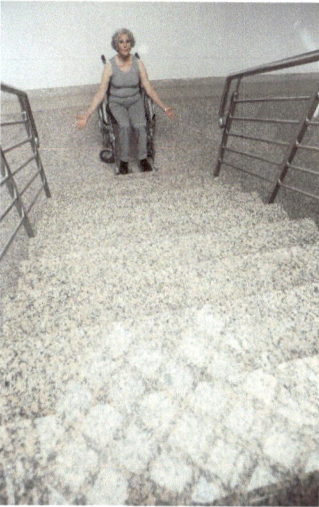

Someone else's experience does not have to be yours! Sometimes all the external information and expectations are overwhelming, and might make you feel that managing your pain is not possible at all.

Childbirth is a good example of how a woman's perception of pain can be externally influenced. Marie Mongan, birthing expert and author of *HypnoBirthing*, talks of cultures in the world that have their babies in the field, hand them off to the midwife, and go back to work. Pain is simply not a big part of birthing their babies. In contrast, the birthing process is a billion-dollar industry in the United States. Mothers and grandmothers love to tell the horror stories of their labor, and these ideas have become deeply embedded In our modern-day culture. The pain of labor can also become a badge of courage and strength. "Oh, you think that was bad? My labor lasted eighteen hours, *and* I had back labor with continuous contractions!"

I'll give you a personal example of how the expectation of pain once affected me. I've had quite a few surgeries in my life, and ten years ago I had shoulder surgery. It was a day surgery - in and out of the hospital within a couple of hours - and my expectation was that it would be a piece of cake. I was told that I only needed a ride home because of the anesthesia. The doctor gave me a prescription for a thirty-day supply of OxyContin. I asked the pharmacist to fill only six pills of the prescription, and I was doubtful I would even take that many. I was so confidant that this was going to be an easy surgery that I even made plans to go out with friends a few days after the surgery.

As she was preparing the IV, the nurse asked me if I had filled my pain prescription. I told her I had gotten six pills. She looked up from her chart, and I'll never forget what she said as she wrote on the prescription pad. "I'm going to give this to your daughter to get filled while you are in surgery. You will need every one of these. This is a very painful procedure and people always underestimate it because they don't have to spend the night in a hospital."

I entered a state of tangible fear, and those words took on a very real power. In the days following the surgery, I took every one of the thirty pills and then asked my doctor for another two-week supply. I slept on the sofa for two months where I could totally immobilize my arm because the pain would wake me up if my arm moved during the night. Rehab was incredibly painful, and I have never regained a full range of motion in my shoulder. Even compared to my previous back surgery that cut into my spine and left a ten-inch scar, my shoulder surgery was the most painful surgery I have ever had. Talk about hypnotic suggestion! That nurse told me what I would feel, and it manifested in every way I could imagine it would.

The surgeon who performed my knee replacements told me he thought I was making the right decision by doing both my knees at once. When he followed that comforting comment with, "Of course you'll probably cuss my name for the next six months," I called a colleague for a session to get that thought out of my subconscious mind!

The negative thoughts you think, and the words you say to yourself and hear from others can be powerful suggestions to your subconscious mind, affecting your body in negative ways. They can trigger feelings and behaviors you don't like. They can start to define you.

It's often that clients with chronic pain say they *always* have some level of pain. Typically this is not really true. When I ask if they have pain while relaxing in the tub or shower, or when they've slept for five hours straight, or when they are watching television or having dinner with friends, they realize there *are* times that the pain isn't ruining or controlling their life completely. It is this kind of awareness that kindles hope, and together we can start to affect change.

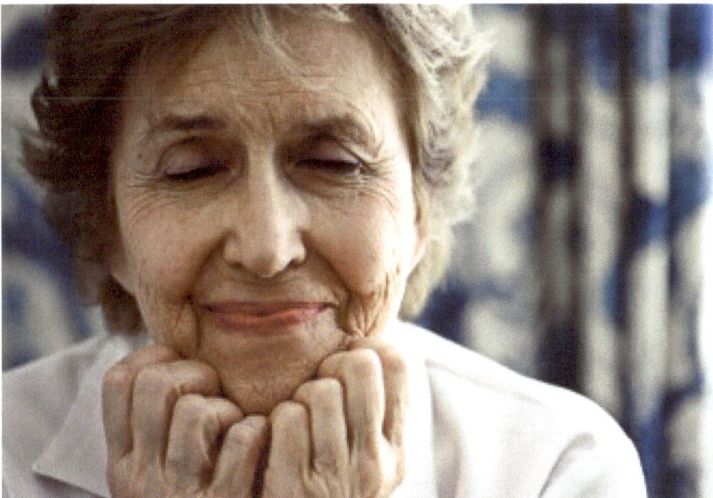

Working with Clients

I only work with pain clients if they have a referral from their doctor. This is extremely important, as sometimes pain serves a purpose. If the pain serves a necessary purpose, I teach the client to turn it down, not eliminate it. This provides a level of comfort that allows them to live their lives to the fullest capacity.

It is my practice to thoroughly understand what is going on with a client. Sometimes the doctor can give me a more complete understanding. I may have questions about a medication the client is taking and if it could have an effect on the depth of his or her trance state. At times, I may also want to hear how the doctor has expressed the client's condition and prognosis. I may need to "de-program" some suggestions that the doctor may have unintentionally made that could interfere with the client's recovery and expectations for the future. And of course, I always tell a prospective client that it is only with the permission of his or her doctor that any elimination or change in medication should be made, or any new activity should be added to their routine.

I also like to communicate with doctors because it gives me the opportunity to educate them. They get to see that hypnosis can really make a difference for their patients. This is how I work to affect change within the current system. It is how you can, too. If you have had success with hypnosis in stopping smoking, managing your pain, improving your sleep or reducing stress, or losing weight - tell your doctor. Doctors can't learn about the benefits of hypnosis if we don't let them know.

There are many techniques that I use when helping clients manage their pain. The reasoning behind the use of any given technique depends on the type of pain (acute or chronic), where it is located, how it manifests, the type of client, and much, much more. Sometimes I have to experiment with several ideas to see what resonates the strongest and gives the most relief.

Words and expectations are very important. Beginning at the first visit, I have the client change their language, and start to refer to pain as discomfort. No one likes pain but everyone can handle a little discomfort. I stress that the client should focus on their level of *comfort*.

Setting the client's goals, and listing the benefits they will experience when they have achieved the level of comfort they desire, are the most important parts of the preparation for their sessions. For example, a client may say that she wants more flexibility. If we further define that goal and determine how flexibility would make a difference in her life (for example, because she will be able to get on the floor and play with her grandchildren) that goal becomes more powerful and motivating than simply wanting to be flexible!

I also spend time talking about what the pain feels like for the client. I ask, "What would you have to do to *me* to cause me to feel what you feel?" Once I have a good handle on the negative sensation, I want to know what she would *like* to feel, or what she thinks will change the feeling into something pleasant.

Hypnosis focuses on the positive. Remember, what you focus on expands. Those with chronic pain have focused on the negative for so long that the pain has become who they *are*. Providing a picture of hope and possibility is critical, and so is changing their self-talk.

The clients who get the best results have a few elements in common: they really want the change, they practice the techniques I teach them on a regular basis, and they learn and practice self-hypnosis. If they do these things they won't need me for very long.

As I've stated previously, the brain cannot tell the difference between what's real and what is vividly imagined. I may use an approach the client has already found to be successful, for example, a shot or medicine that numbed the painful area. Or I'll use a few techniques that I find to work with most clients. My favorites have everything to do with how the body and mind can work together in a natural organic way. Here is the secret to how I managed my post - surgical pain after my bilateral knee replacement. I simply used my breath. Before I talk about the power of the breath, it's important to understand a little about how your body works.

Your Autonomic Nervous System

You get stressed. You calm down. The part of your nervous system that controls this, that is designed to keep you in homeostasis or in balance, is called the Autonomic Nervous System (ANS). It is made up of two separate parts: the Sympathetic Nervous System (SNS) and the Parasympathetic Nervous System (PNS). I keep these two straight by remembering that *para*chutes let you down gently - and so the *Para*sympathetic Nervous System is the one that calms you.

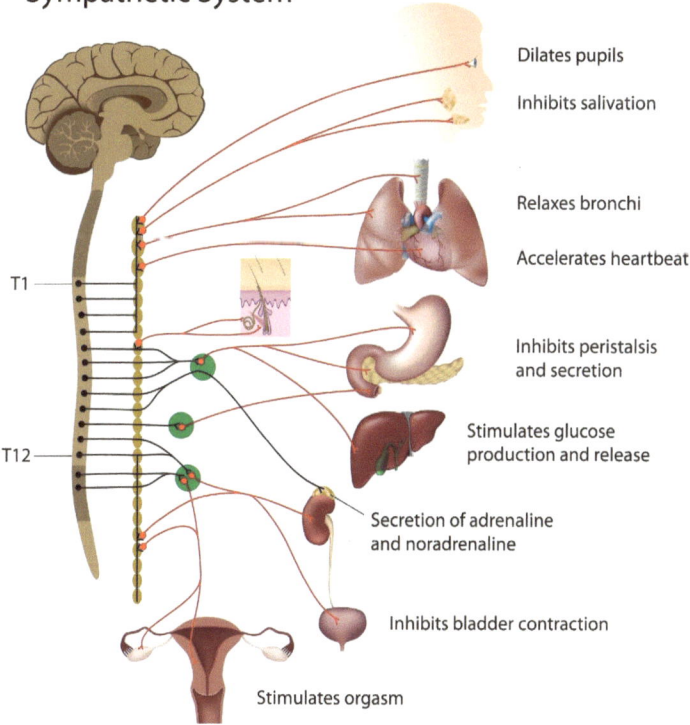

Sympathetic System

Dilates pupils

Inhibits salivation

Relaxes bronchi

Accelerates heartbeat

Inhibits peristalsis and secretion

Stimulates glucose production and release

Secretion of adrenaline and noradrenaline

Inhibits bladder contraction

Stimulates orgasm

T1

T12

The SNS is the part that produces adrenaline and cortisol, the flight-or-fight chemicals in your body. These chemicals enable you to jump out of the way of a swerving car, that keeps you alert if you are in a strange neighborhood late at night, or cause you to duck when that foul ball comes flying into the stands. Stress chemicals cause your nerves to activate nociception pathways (danger messages) that can cause your brain to send pain in your body.

Parasympathetic System

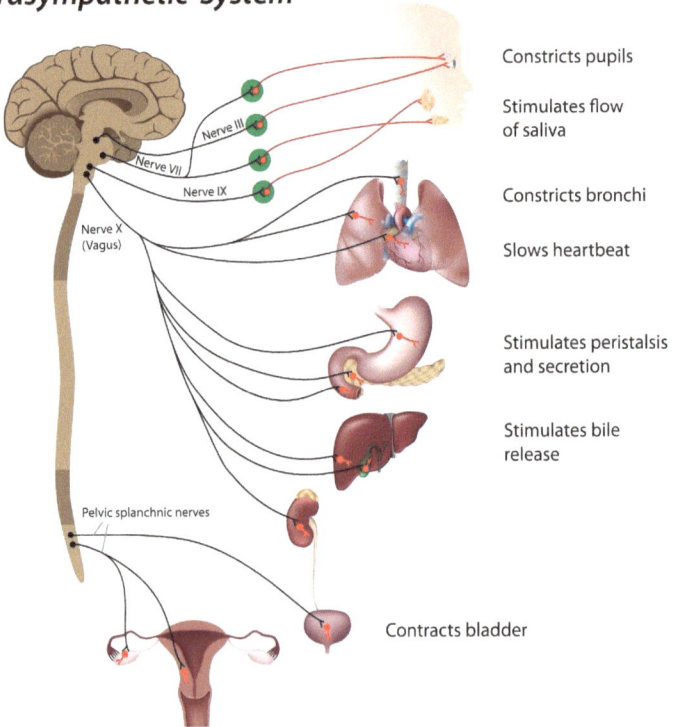

Constricts pupils

Stimulates flow of saliva

Constricts bronchi

Slows heartbeat

Stimulates peristalsis and secretion

Stimulates bile release

Contracts bladder

Nerve III
Nerve VII
Nerve IX
Nerve X (Vagus)
Pelvic splanchnic nerves

The PNS is the part that produces chemicals that calm you down, such as endorphins, serotonin and melatonin. These natural, feel-good chemicals compare to their manufactured drug counterparts Morphine, Ambien and Xanax. But they are fifty times more powerful than the synthetic versions.

The longest nerve in your body is the vagus nerve. It comes directly from your brain stem and is one of the most important parts of your nervous system, touching most of your major organs along the way toward the lower part of your body. It sends and receives messages to and from your brain. Some of the main functions of the vagus nerve include regulating your breath and speech, monitoring and regulating your heartbeat, informing your brain that you are ingesting food, that digestion is complete, and that the gastric region needs to be emptied of food. It also is important in stimulating the parasympathetic nervous system (PNS).

In an article in Psychology Today, Christopher Bergland said that, "The vagus nerve is the commander-in-chief when it comes to having grace under pressure. The sympathetic nervous system is geared to rev you up like the gas pedal in an automobile – it thrives on adrenaline and cortisol and is part of the fight-or-flight response. The parasympathetic nervous system is the polar opposite. The vagus nerve is command central for the function of your parasympathetic nervous system."[35]

When you are in pain, your sympathetic nervous system is highly engaged and it is harder to relax and feel calm. The "tighter" you get, the more you feel the pain. One of the ways to turn down the volume on pain is to activate the parasympathetic nervous system. The function of the vagus nerve at the base of your diaphragm is to send a signal to your brain to stimulate the parasympathetic nervous system and bring your body back into balance. This is why your breath is so powerful in managing stress and pain. Proper breathing stimulates the vagus nerve. Your brain cannot produce adrenaline and cortisol at the same time it releases endorphins and other calming chemicals. These calming chemicals from the parasympathetic nervous system are released and the sympathetic nervous system is quieted, naturally relieving your pain.

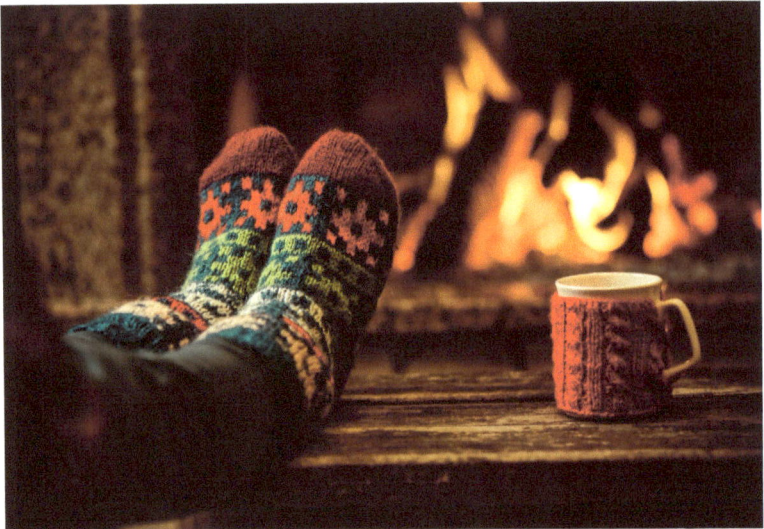

It's All in Your Imagination

Some of you may have been told by your doctor that your pain is in your head, or that it is just in your imagination. While there is some truth to that, the pain can still be manifesting in your body. The good news is that you can use your imagination to turn down the volume or get rid of your pain completely, by using hypnosis.

I cannot state often enough that the brain can't tell the difference between what is real and what is vividly imagined. When you engage your imagination, using as many of your senses and feelings as possible, your brain acts as though it is actually happening. Your thoughts become real. And you can choose those thoughts wisely.

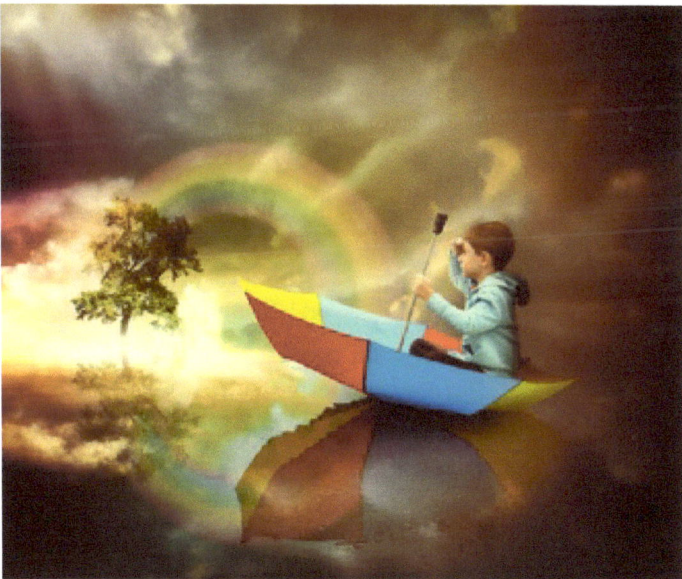

Imagination can be engaged in pain management in a variety of ways. With some clients I might use metaphor - imagining the pain shrinking from the size of a beach ball to a ping-pong ball that you could put in your pocket, and hardly notice it at all. Or perhaps you can visualize the pain shrinking down to the tiniest little object, place it in a box, and put it away on a very high shelf where it gets dusty and forgotten. There are literally hundreds of metaphors to be used and they are limited only by your imagination.

I've also mentioned the importance and power of shifting your focus. Perhaps there was a time when you were very hungry. Just as you were searching the kitchen for something to eat, the phone rang. After two or three minutes on the phone, with your attention totally diverted, you hang up and have forgotten that you were hungry. Shifting your focus to something other than your pain can accomplish this exact thing. And it only takes a couple of minutes of distraction to create a different, automated response.

Finding your "happy place" is one way of shifting focus and taking back control over pain. In that place, nothing bothers or disturbs you, and you are completely comfortable and relaxed. Some clients have so much pain that they say they don't have a happy place. In these cases, I ask them to imagine what a happy place would be like if this place *did* exist. In hypnosis, we can create this place together, in great detail. This place is a safe space where only comfort is experienced. Once you realize this is possible,
It is.

Just Breathe

There are many techniques that hypnotists use with clients to help them deal with their issues. I have a toolbox full of techniques to use in pain management. The tools I choose and the new ones I create can be very specific to each client. But there is one technique I

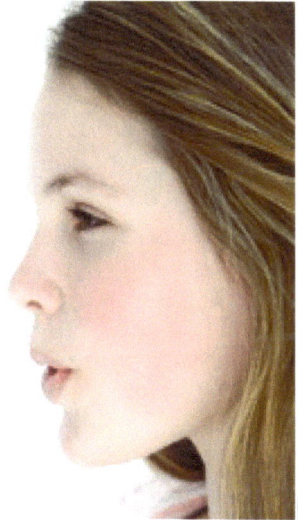

consistently teach my clients for stress and pain relief: the power of the breath.

Your breath is by far one of the most effective techniques there is for managing pain. It is completely natural, costs you nothing, and has no negative side effects. It works because it is how your body is *designed* to work. You were born with this skill; you just haven't learned how to use it to your best advantage.

What do you tell someone who is stressed or really

upset, or who's just hurt themselves? "Relax! Take a deep breath!" You say it intuitively because you know it works. Now you know the biological reason why.

Taking a deep breath in, holding it for a count of two, then exhaling it slowly, causes the vagus nerve to be naturally stimulated. Holding for a count of two allows for the full exchange of oxygen and carbon dioxide.

There is a second step to the breathing technique that I teach that is significant. Because what you focus on expands, you shift your focus from the pain to something else. With the breath, you shift to a state of relaxation and control. As you exhale, you count in your mind from fast to slow, loud to soft: 5,4,3,2,1, followed by the word "relax." Doing this five times in a row allows the vagus nerve to be naturally stimulated and for you to shift your focus from the pain to a state of relaxation by giving yourself the suggestion using the word "relax" every time you breathe.

Using this simple technique is how I managed my pain after undergoing bilateral knee replacement. My breath was my most effective weapon in combating pain. For two months before surgery, I practiced this technique at least five times a day, five breaths in a row. I substituted the word "relax" for "total comfort." That's it!

It takes five to seven weeks for the brain to automate a physical response for something to become a habit. When the day of my surgery came, I only had to start to take a breath and my brain knew exactly what I wanted - total comfort. My brain connected the expectation of comfort with my breath as the trigger. The manner of the breath, the counting, all became associated with my goal of comfort. FARE - Focus, Associate, Repeat, Expect!

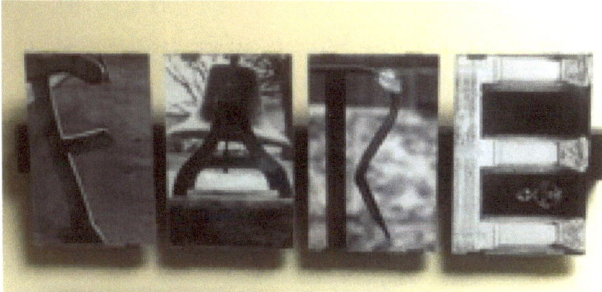

Focus - Associate - Repeat - Expect

While this concept seems so simple, it is exactly how your mind and body are created to work together. Just as you no longer have to think about how to tie your shoes or how to brush your teeth, you can train your brain to produce a sensation in your body that you desire, simply by using the natural biology of your body and mind.

Success Stories

I'd like to share a few success stories:
A client was preparing for a bilateral mastectomy. She had a lot of emotion and worry around the procedure. I gave her simple suggestions and reaffirmed her belief that she was making the right decision for herself. She listened to a recording where she imagined, step-by-step, how wonderful the surgery and recovery would be. She practiced self-hypnosis daily for two weeks before her surgery. After the surgery, my client had very little discomfort, took minimal pain medication, and was told by her doctor that she had never seen a patient come through the surgery so easily.

Another client had an operation for hammertoes on both of her feet. She did not have general anesthesia; instead, they sedated her heavily with medication. While being prepped for the surgery, she used self-hypnosis, giving herself instructions to stay in trance for two hours, feeling totally relaxed. Unfortunately, they started the surgery late, and before they were done, she recalls hearing the anesthesiologist say, "She's waking up." She immediately put herself back into trance and awoke later in the recovery room. This experience helped her realize just how much control she has!

Six weeks later, when the pins were removed from her toes, she focused on staying completely comfortable and having minimal bleeding during the procedure in her doctor's office. He was amazed to see the results!
The same client also suffered from Restless Leg Syndrome (RLS). RLS worsens with inactivity. She was

instructed to keep her feet elevated for six weeks after the surgery. She was worried about her legs twitching. I suggested that she practice her self-hypnosis daily and imagine doing physical activity. She understood that if she vividly imagined doing an activity, her brain would react as if she was *actually* doing it. In trance, I had her imagine doing some of her favorite hobbies, and then she regularly practiced the techniques in self-hypnosis. The RLS was not a factor during her recovery.

Another client suffers from fibromyalgia. She begins experiencing pain in her neck and shoulders first, and then the pain spreads down into her chest and body, typically in the early afternoon while working. Her pain interfered greatly with her work, and sometimes causes her to be unable to drive home. She is extremely sensitive to touch, to the extent that even having sheets touch her body could be extremely uncomfortable. We spent time managing her stress and I gave her multiple suggestions for how she would rather feel. She is now able to perceive her discomfort in a different way and turn down the volume on any other sensations.

A man with chronic back pain was able to produce "glove anesthesia," a numbing of his hand through suggestion. I then taught him how to transfer that numbness to his back. He does this by himself while practicing self-hypnosis every day, and his quality of life has improved dramatically.

A former client suffered from daily headaches for over five years. Her doctor had told her there was nothing else he could do for her, as arthritis and stenosis in her neck caused the pain. He said the pain served no purpose so it would be appropriate to eliminate it using hypnosis. This client had previous success with a shot in her head that numbed the entire area, though it only lasted 24 hours. I used the suggestion of that same medication, given in a pleasant way, to shrink the inflamed nerves down to a size so small that it ceased to bother or disturb her. She continues to use that imagery every day in her happy place when she practices her self-hypnosis and remains free of headaches.

A current client is an elderly woman who is in tremendous pain from multiple surgeries. She is no longer able to take her opioids and was referred by a pain clinic that had no other options to offer her. When she arrived at our center, she was crying due to the pain she was experiencing. Getting up and down was so painful that Linda, one of our hypnotists, conducted the session in her wheelchair. She left with her comfort level at a 2 (with 0 being total comfort). The second week she came in with an additional issue - shingles. Linda continued working with techniques for her discomfort. She also began the process of releasing pent-up anger that was contributing to her pain level. (Remember, the brain processes emotional pain in the same way as physical pain.) Last week she arrived all dressed up, hair and makeup done, using her walker and laughing. She is amazed at her progress. She practices her self-hypnosis every day. When this client first visited our center she was ready to give up because the pain was making her life unbearable. In three short weeks her life has completely changed.

All of these clients had run out of hope. Everything they had tried had failed to get the results they were seeking. The outcomes that these clients have achieved are why I am a hypnotist. If you would have told me that hypnosis was transformational at the time I knew nothing about it, I would probably have laughed and walked away. But today, many clients later, I am hard pressed to find a more suitable word than "transformational" to describe what can happen for a client!

Pain may be inevitable, but suffering is certainly an option. You can choose, one way or another.

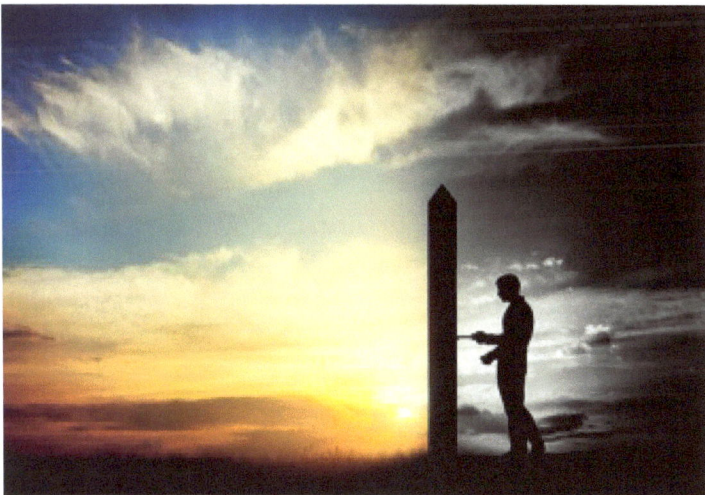

Pain Studies on the Efficacy of Hypnosis

The research on using hypnosis for pain relief covers a broad spectrum of applications from acute pain to post-surgical pain to chronic conditions. There has also been research that indicates that hypnosis is helpful for a variety of medical conditions, like Irritable Bowel Syndrome, warts, burns and nausea. As promised, here is more research that confirms the benefits of hypnosis for pain relief.

In a study using pain stimulation by pinprick and laser heat, direct suggestions given in hypnosis resulted in a significant decrease in pain.[29]

As previously mentioned, the mechanism of analgesia (the ability to only feel "a little something") from hypnosis appears to differ significantly from a placebo effect and from induced endorphin production (similar to the effects of morphine). Naloxone, a drug that "reverses" the effects of an opiate like heroin or morphine, does not block the pain relief that was achieved through hypnosis. In one study, pain was produced in volunteers by tightly inflating a blood pressure cuff on the upper arm, followed by exercise. The cuff was left on for ten minutes. Before hypnosis, all participants reported a pain level of 8 or more (with 10 being the most intense). While in hypnosis, all reported a pain level of 0, and this relief was *not* altered substantially by administration of naloxone.[36] This demonstrates that the suggestion to not have pain continued to produce relief from the pain, even though the Naloxone would have neutralized the endorphins, allowing the pain to be felt.

In the clinical setting, hypnosis for pain relief appears to have similar benefit. In a randomized, double blind study for the use of Naloxone, patients with neuropathic pain (a chronic pain state usually caused by tissue injury) were taught self-hypnosis. Considerable relief from pain was achieved with hypnosis, and this relief was not reversed by administration of Naloxone. In patients with low hypnotizability, hypnosis was equal to placebo for pain relief, whereas highly hypnotizable people benefited more from hypnosis than from placebo. This finding indicates that hypnosis involves at least two effects: a placebo-type effect and one in which suggestion actually distorts perception.[28,37]

A meta-analysis published in 2000 evaluated the use of hypnosis for pain relief from eighteen studies conducted during the preceding twenty years. This review indicated that hypnosis offered a moderate to large analgesic effect for many types of pain, which met "the criteria for well established treatment." Because hypnosis was noted to benefit most patients, a broader application of its use was advocated. A comprehensive review of hypnosis for pain relief published in 2003 found hypnosis to be superior to placebo for acute pain, and at times superior to pain relief achieved by other means. It was concluded that hypnosis for chronic pain is a viable option, with the understanding that pain therapy requires "multi-dimensional assessment and treatment."[31,38]

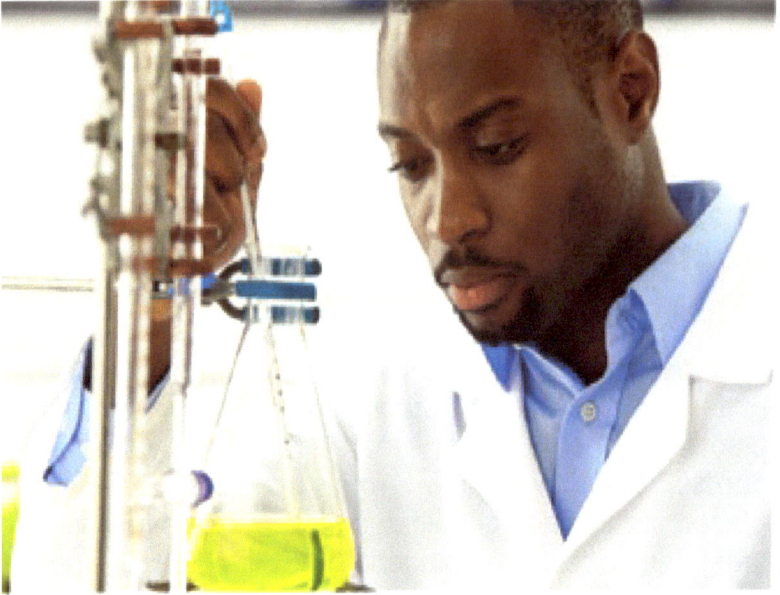

This brings me to another significant point. Hypnosis is classified by many states as alternative medicine. Hypnosis can be effective in and of itself, but it isn't a matter of using only "this" method of treatment or only using hypnosis. I view hypnosis as *complementary* to other methods of treatment for pain. Hypnosis is highly effective when combined with other alternative modalities and/or conventional medicine.

Choosing a Hypnotist

Hypnosis is regulated in many states, but not licensed. Traditionally, insurance does not pay; however, a few insurance companies have been known to cover hypnosis if a medical doctor prescribes it. Ask your doctor and call your insurance company.

I would be remiss if I didn't give you advice on how to choose a hypnosis practitioner. Ask the practitioner about their training, and even if they are a doctor or a therapist, ask how often they use hypnosis in their practice. Doctors and therapists may be well qualified in their profession, but some may not be as well versed in hypnosis. Hypnosis is not a part of traditional training in medical and psychological fields. I find many who use hypnosis as a tool in their practice have only taken a weekend course. It is my professional opinion that this is not sufficient. Anyone can learn to induce hypnosis with a willing participant and a YouTube video. The important part is in understanding what to do once a person is in trance. Training and practice are very important!

Here are important criteria you should look for in any hypnotist and his or her practice:

- Be sure the practitioner has taken their practical training at a licensed school, preferably in a live class versus an online program.
- 100 hours of class time should be the minimum hours of training.
- Ask what kind of hypnosis is practiced - direct suggestion or regression, Ericksonian or Elman.

If they are well-trained in both that's even better!
- Are they members of a well-established organization that has a code of ethics and standards of practice for their training and for their members?
- Ask if they are required to take continuing education to maintain their certification.
- Research. Research. Research. Remember that anyone can make themselves look like a professional with a good website. Be a responsible consumer and check them out.
- Ask for a consultation and make sure they are a good fit for you, in philosophy and in personality.
- Ask if they provide a Client Bill of Rights, a document that discloses their office practices and fees, and your rights as a client.
- Ask if they have experience in working with your issue.
- If they promise guaranteed results, pass. They cannot guarantee your success!

The National Guild of Hypnotists is a good place to start to find a practitioner in your area (NGH.net). You can also visit my website at **www.FAREHypnosis.com**, or send me an email. I'm happy to guide you.

If you are considering a career in hypnosis, or want to add hypnotism to your current skill set, a quality school is essential. Here are some questions to ask about the school you might choose:

- Is the school licensed by the state or otherwise legally operating?
- With what hypnosis organization are you training

or certifying?
- Do they provide ongoing support after graduation?
- Do you receive supervised practice?
- Do they offer advice about setting up a practice?
- Can you retake the course for free?
- What are the instructor's qualifications and are they still seeing clients?
- Are there non-hypnosis topics included? (Avoid these)
- How large are the classes? (Should be less than 20)
- What kind of issues will you be able to work with upon graduating?
- How systemized is the approach?

Parting Thoughts

Is hypnosis the right modality for *your* pain? I can't say without a thorough consultation to what extent hypnosis can help you manage your pain. Every person, and every situation, is different. Most of my clients have positive results using hypnosis. Success is directly related to the amount of effort the client puts into the process, and how diligently he or she practices their self-hypnosis.

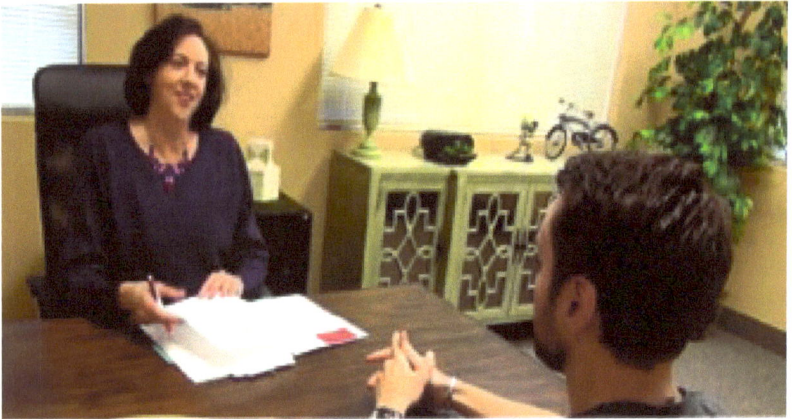

I have even had a few clients (though it is rare) leave my office after the first visit with very little discomfort and never have their pain return. The majority of my clients have the results that they are seeking within four to six visits. They continue to have success in managing their pain by using self-hypnosis.

The case to be made for using hypnosis for pain management is simply this:
- No negative side effects
- No pills or implanted devices

- Minimal investment
- Relatively fast results
- Self-care
- No ongoing expense once the techniques are learned

Most of my clients come to me after having tried everything else and nothing has worked. My goal at my Center is for people to think of using hypnosis as part of their *first* steps, and to complement other treatments that they might already be using.

Tackling the opioid problem begins with each one of us doing our part. You can help in spreading the word so others realize that they, too, can take back control over their pain. Share this book with your doctor, friend or family member to let them know they have alternative options for their pain management.

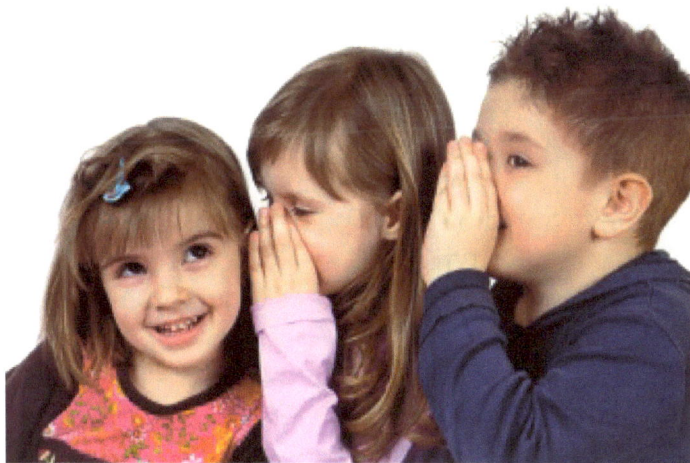

About the Author

Roberta Fernandez, BCH, CPHI
Board Certified Hypnotist
Certified Professional Hypnosis Instructor

Roberta is the Founder and President of The FARE Hypnosis Center in Eden Prairie, Minnesota.

She is certified:

- By the National Guild of Hypnotists as a Board Certified Hypnotist
- By the National Guild of Hypnotists as a Certified Instructor
- By the National Guild of Hypnotists' Complementary Medical Certification
- As a Certified Professional Hypnosis Instructor (CPHI) by the Banyan Hypnosis Center in California
- As a 5-Path Consulting Hypnotist and 7th Path® Self Hypnosis Teacher by the Banyan Hypnosis Center in California
- In Pain Management from the American School of Clinical Hypnosis, International
- As an NLP Master Practitioner and Consulting Hypnotist and by the Minnesota Institute of Advanced Communication Skills
- As a Hypnotic Gastric Band Surgery Specialist, by Anthony F. DeMarco, PhD
- As a Golf Specialist by Laura Boynton King, under the auspices of the NGH
- By The Mottin and Johnson Institute in Pain Management

Roberta has 30 years of experience in education, training, sustainability and finance, working across public and private sectors. Past clients include Kemps, Pentair, Sam's Club, Starwood VO, JP Morgan Chase, the DNR, and many other government and educational institutions.

She is her own "walking" testimonial, having used hypnosis to successfully manage her severe knee pain pre-surgery, and after a bilateral knee replacement. She used only hypnosis instead of drugs to manage her pain, and she experienced no pain.

At the time of this printing, Roberta is currently using hypnosis for weight loss and has lost thirty pounds. She practices The 7th Path® Self Hypnosis program on a daily basis.

She uses hypnosis to help others become positive, productive and purposeful in achieving their life goals.

You can contact Roberta at www.FAREHypnosis.com.

To download a complimentary personal relaxation recording to ease your stress, visit: **www.FAREHypnosis.com** Click on the **Downloads and Signup** tab

Citations

1 American Academy of Pain Medicine. Available at http://www.painmed.org/patientcenter/facts_on_pain.as px#burden

2 Centers for Disease Control and Prevention. Increases in Drug and Opioid Overdose Deaths — United States, 2000–2014. MMWR 2015; 64;1-5.

3 Centers for Disease Control and Prevention. Morbidity and Mortality Weekly Report. Available at http://www.cdc.gov/mmwr/preview/mmwrhtml/mm6043 a4.htm?

4 National Centers for Health Statistics. Chartbook on Trends in the Health of Americans 2006, Special Feature: Pain. Available at http://www.cdc.gov/nchs/data/hus/hus06.pdf

5 Centers for Disease Control and Prevention. Morbidity and Mortality Weekly Report. Available at http://www.cdc.gov/mmwr/preview/mmwrhtml/mm6043 a4.htm?s_cid=mm6043a4_w#fig2

6 Chang, H., Daubresse, M., Kruszewski, S., & Alexander, G.C (2014). Prevalence and treatment of pain in emergency departments in the United States, 2000 to 2010. *American Journal of Emergency Medicine*; 32(5): 421-431.

7 Daubresse, M., Chang, H., Yu, Y., Viswanathan, S., Shah, N.D., Stafford, R.S., ...Alexander, G.C. (2013). Ambulatory diagnosis and treatment of nonmalignant

pain in the United States, 2000 to 2010. *Medical Care*; 51(10): 870-878.

8 Results from the 2009 National Survey on Drug Use and Health (NSDUH): National Findings, SAMHSA (2010).
9 2010 Monitoring the Future, University of Michigan. Available at http://monitoringthefuture.org/

10 Substance Abuse and Mental Health Services Administration, Center for Behavioral Health Statistics and Quality (2015). Behavioral health trends in the United States: Results from the 2014 National Survey on Drug Use and Health. Available at http://www.samhsa.gov/data/sites/default/files/NSDUH-FRR1-2014/NSDUH-FRR1-2014.pdf.

11 Hedegaard, H., Chen, L.H., & Warner, M. (2015). Drug-Poisoning Deaths Involving Heroin: United States, 2000-2013 (No. 190). US Department of Health and Human Services, Centers for Disease Control and Prevention, National Center for Health Statistics.

12 Cicero, T.J., Ellis, M.S., Surratt, H.L., & Kurtz, S.P. (2014). The changing face of heroin use in the United States: a retrospective analysis of the past 50 years. *JAMA Psychiatry*,71(7):821-826.

13 Centers for Disease Control and Prevention (2014). Opioid Painkiller Prescribing, Where You Live Makes a Difference. Available at http://www.cdc.gov/vitalsigns/opioid-prescribing/

14 Grace, P.M., Strand, K.A., Galer, E.L., Urban, D.J.,

Wang, X., Baratta, M.V., ... Watkins, L.R. (2016). Morphine paradoxically prolongs neuropathic pain in rats by amplifying spinal NLRP3 inflammasome activation. *Proceedings of the National Academy of Sciences*; 113(24): E3441-50.

15 Committee on Advancing Pain Research, Care, and Education; National Academies Institute of Medicine (2011). *Relieving Pain in America, A Blueprint for Transforming Prevention, Care, Education and Research.* The National Academies Press.
16 Coalition Against Insurance Fraud (2007). Prescription for peril: how insurance fraud finances theft and abuse of addictive prescription drugs. Available at http://www.insurancefraud.org/downloads/drugDiversio n.pdf

17 Integrated benefits Institute; Chronic Disease Profile: Low Back Pain; Available at https://ibiweb.org/research-resources/results/.

18 Elman, D. (1964).*Hypnotherapy*; Glendale, CA; Westwood Publishing Co.

19 Spiegel, H., Greenleaf, M., Spiegel, D. (2002). Hypnosis. In Sadock, B.J., & Sadock, V.A., eds. Kaplan & Sadock's *Comprehensive Textbook of Psychiatry, Vol 2. 7th ed.* (pp. 2138-2146). Philadelphia, Pa: Lippincott Williams & Wilkins.

20 Kosslyn, S.M., Thompson, W.L., Costantini-Ferrando, M.F., Alpert, N.M., & Spiegel, D. (2000). Hypnotic visual illusion alters color processing in the brain. *American Journal of Psychiatry*; 157:1279-1284.

21 Koivisto, M., Kirjanen, S., Revonsuo, A., & Kallio, S. (2013). A Preconscious Neural Mechanism of Hypnotically Altered Colors: A Double Case Study. *PLoS ONE;* 8(8): e70900.

22 Tasman, A., Kay, J., & Lieberman, J.A. (1997). *Psychiatry, Vol 2.* Philadelphia, Pa: WB Saunders Co.

23 Banyai, E.I., & Hilgard, E.R. (1976). A comparison of active-alert hypnotic induction with traditional relaxation induction. *Journal of Abnormal Psychology;* 85:218-224.

24 Szechtman, H., Woody, E., Bowers, K.S., & Nahmias, C. (1998). Where the imaginal appears real: a positron emission tomography study of auditory hallucinations. *Proceedings of the National Academy of Sciences*; 95:1956-1960.

25 Yue, G. H., & Cole, K.J. (1992). Strength increases from the motor program: comparison of training with maximal voluntary and imagined muscle contractions. *Journal of Neurophysiology* 67(5):1114-1123.

26 Rainville, P., Hofbauer, R.K., Bushnell, M.C., Duncan, G.H., & Price, D.D. (2002). Hypnosis modulates activity in brain structures involved in the regulation of consciousness. *Journal of Cognitive Neuroscience*; 14:887-901.

27 Jensen, S.M., Barabasz, A., Barabasz, M., Warner, D. (2001). EEG P300 event-related markers of hypnosis. *American Journal of Clinical Hypnosis*;44:127-139.

28 McGlashan, T.H., Evans, F.J., & Orne, M.T. (1969). The nature of hypnotic analgesia and placebo response to experimental pain. *Psychosomatic* Medicine;31:227-246.

29 Zachariae, R. & Bjerring, P. (1990). The effect of hypnotically induced analgesia on flare reaction of the cutaneous histamine prick test. *Archives of Dermatological Research*;282:539-543.

30 Spiegel, D., Bierre, P., & Rootenberg, J. (1989). Hypnotic alteration of somatosensory perception. *American Journal of Psychiatry*;146:749-754.

31 Patterson, D.R. & Jensen, M.P. (2003). Hypnosis and clinical pain. *Psychological Bulletin*;129:495-521.

32 Lipton, B.H. (2008). *Biology of Belief.*Hay House Publications.

33 Banyan, C. D. (2003).*The Secret Language of Feelings.* St. Paul, MN: Abbott Publishing House, Inc.

34 Louw, A. & Puentedura, E. (2013). *Therapeutic Neuroscience Education:Teaching Patients About Pain;.* International Spine and Institute.

35 Bergland, Christopher (2013, February). *The* Neurobiology of Grace Under Pressure. *Psychology Today,* Available at https://www.psychologytoday.com/blog/the-athletes-way/201302/the-neurobiology-grace-under-pressure

36 Goldstein, A. & Hilgard, E.R. (1975). Failure of the

opiate antagonist naloxone to modify hypnotic analgesia. *Proceedings of the National Academy of Sciences*; 72:2041-2043.

37   Spiegel, D. & Albert, L.H. (1983). Naloxone fails to reverse hypnotic alleviation of chronic pain. *Psychopharmacology*; 81:140-143.

38   Montgomery, G.H., DuHamel, K.N. &Redd, W.H., A meta-analysis of hypnotically induced analgesia: how effective is hypnosis? *Int J Clin Exp Hypn*; 48:138-153.

www.ingramcontent.com/pod-product-compliance
Lightning Source LLC
Chambersburg PA
CBHW040513290326
41930CB00036B/111